AAS
Agents and Actions Supplements
Vol. 32

Series Editor
K. Brune, Erlangen

Birkhäuser Verlag
Basel · Boston · Berlin

Drugs in Inflammation

Edited by

Michael J. Parnham
Michael A. Bray
Wim B. van den Berg

1991

Birkhäuser Verlag
Basel · Boston · Berlin

Volume Editors' Addresses:

M. J. Parnham
Parnham Advisory Services
Hankelstrasse 43
D–W– 5300 Bonn
formerly of Nattermann
& Cie. GmbH, Cologne, FRG

M. A. Bray
Ciba-Geigy AG
R 1056. 215

CH – 4002 Basel
Switzerland

W. B. van den Berg
Dept. of Rheumatology
University Hospital

NL – 6525 GA Nijmegen
The Netherlands

Deutsche Bibliothek Cataloging-in-Publication Data

Drugs in inflammation / ed. by Michael J. Parnham ... – Basel ;
Boston ; Berlin : Birkhäuser, 1991
(Agents and actions : Supplements ; Vol. 32)
ISBN 3-7643-2504-6 (Basel ...)
ISBN 0-8176-2504-6 (Boston)
NE: Parnham, Michael J. [Hrsg.]; Agents and actions / Supplements

Printed in Germany on acid-free paper from the authors' camera-ready manuscripts
ISBN 3-7643-2504-6
ISBN 0-8176-2504-6

TABLE OF CONTENTS

PREFACE

On June 28-29, 1990 in Noordwijk, The Netherlands, the International Association of Inflammation Societies (IAIS) organized their first symposium on Drugs in Inflammation. The symposium was an official satellite of the IXth International Congress of Pharmacology (IUPHAR). This volume contains the proceedings from this satellite meeting.

The IAIS was constituted in 1988 when representatives of the Inflammation Research Association (IRA), European Workshop on Inflammation (EWI) and British Inflammation Research Association (BIRAs) met at White Haven, Pennsylvania during the Fourth International Conference of the IRA and the group decided that improved communication between inflammation societies could be achieved by establishment of a society. The IAIS would encourage and foster collaboration between the many inflammation societies throughout the world and assist in the establishment of new societies whenever possible.

The satellite was a major success thanks to the efforts of the planning committee: Wim van den Berg, the local organizer, Mike Bray, the programme chairman, Rodger McMillan, Greg Harper, Mike Parnham and Kay Brune. In addition, the chairman and presenters ensured the scientific content of the meeting was of a very high standard. Most importantly, the 100 participants from 15 countries made the sessions lively and interactive.

The IAIS will hopefully organize additional symposiums in the future.

Alan J. Lewis, Ph.D.
Chairman, IAIS

Reducing the Side-Effects of Anti-Inflammatory Drugs

AAS 32
Drugs in Inflammation

TOWARDS SAFER NONSTEROIDAL ANTI-INFLAMMATORY DRUGS

K. Brune and W.S. Beck

Department of Pharmacology, University of Erlangen-Nuernberg, Universitaetsstrasse 22, 8520 Erlangen, F.R.G.

SUMMARY: More than one hundred years ago salicylic acid and its salts were introduced into the therapy of rheumatic diseases. Ninety years ago aspirin was discovered, and within the last forty years phenylbutazone, indomethacin, ibuprofen, the oxicams and many others were discovered. All of these drugs are acidic. They inhibit the prostaglandin synthetase, combine analgesic and anti-inflammatory activity and show side-effects mainly in the GI-tract, liver, bone-marrow, and kidney. Within the last twenty years, however, distinct relationships between effects and side-effects could be shown:

1. Rapid absorption beginning in the stomach goes along with intensive gastric-duodenal irritation and ulceration.
2. A high degree of enterohepatic circulation appears to be associated with ileal and jejunal ulcerations and perforations.
3. Intensive hepatic metabolisation may be related to enhanced hepatic damage.
4. Intensive intrarenal circulation of the active moiety may be related to kidney damage.

These observations indicate that certain pharmacokinetic characteristics of distinct nonsteroidal anti-inflammatory drugs (NSAIDs) are responsible, at least in part, for well-known side-effects. It is obvious that modifying the pharmacokinetics of the active principle may reduce specific types of side-effects. The clinical success of these attempts are limited but altogether promising.

INTRODUCTION

The ancient greek and roman physicians, as well as the famous Hildegard of Bingen and the Reverend E. Stone, used extracts of willow bark in order to treat inflammation, inflammatory pain, gout and other ailments. They complained that these extracts were not always effective and that they caused gastric and intestinal irritation and diarrhea (Collier, 1984). The first improvement of willow bark extracts was achieved when Piria, Kolbe and von Heyden isolated salicylic acid and its first salts, and started mass production of the effective ingredient, salicylic acid (Rainsford, 1984). The resulting powder, however, was hardly palatable, and many patients suffering from chronic polyarthitis complained about the ugly taste and the resulting aversion against swallowing upto 7 grams of such a powder every day (comp. e.g., Collier, 1984). These complaints from his father urged the chemist, Hoffmann, of the company Bayer, to synthesize esters and other chemical derivatives of salicylic acid. One of them, later on named aspirin, was obviously more palatable to Hoffmann's father. Moreover, it turned out to be less irritant than salicylic acid, at least when administered to the slimy skin of goldfish fins. These pharmacological models (at that time) of human mucosa turned greyish when exposed to the same molar concentration of salicylic acid, but did not change their appearance when exposed to aspirin (Dreser, 1907). The first pharmacologist at Bayer, Dreser, consequently regarded aspirin as a prodrug of salicylic acid which was devoid of some of the unwanted effects of the active ingredient. Probably by ways of misquotation and inadequate translation, aspirin was also believed to be the more potent analgesic and was introduced world-wide as powerful analgesic and antirheumatic drug (Collier, 1984). It was also assumed that it was less toxic than the older salicylic acid (Dreser, 1907). Both claims have to be questioned on the basis of our present knowledge, at least with respect to the analgesic and anti-inflammatory effects of the salicylates

(McCormack and Brune, 1990). It is, however, interesting to realise that the anti-inflammatory analgesic and antipyretic effects of the salicylate molecule were discovered early but also that the unwanted and unpleasant effects of these drugs were recognized early and the two classical ways of amending these problems, namely, producing either molecular modifications or prodrugs of the active ingredient were tried early. As today, the new chemical entity was believed to be better in most respects but later re-investigation caused doubts about these claims. In the following chapters, we shall attempt to show that the same processes have continued for the last ninety years. They have yielded market improvements of the same pharmacological principle. All these improvements appear to be based on findings by serendipity. They may, in retrospect, also be regarded as a logical process taking advantage of improved knowledge and refined research technology.

INCREASING THE POTENCY

One of the main deficits of the early salicylates was their moderate anti-inflammatory action requiring high doses per day. In the early fifties phenylbutazone was discovered by serendipity which proved to be much more potent. Some clinicians believed it is also more efficient in rheumatic diseases. This improvement, however, was paralleled by new forms of toxicity. Phenylbutazone turned out to be equal to aspirin in GI-tract toxicity. However, particularly during long-term treatment, prominent fluid retention due to impaired renal function occurred regulary, and morphological changes in the kidney medulla were occasionally found. Moreover, sudden cardiovascular or central nervous effects occurred during long-term treatment with phenylbutazone (v. Rechenberg, 1957). These latter results were later interpreted as resulting from the slow elimination of phenylbutazone and its major active metabolite, oxyphenbutazone (Brune and Lanz, 1985). Both effects were less pronounced with the next discovery, namely indomethacin. Indomethacin proved to be more potent than phenylbutazone, by that, extending this direction of development. Also kidney damage was less frequent and agranulocytosis and aplastic anemia were not observed. This substance, however, appeared as least as toxic to the GI-tract as phenylbutazone and, in addition, caused central nervous side-effects with great regularity (comp. e.g., Kurowski, 1990). These observations prompted us to speculate why all known, up to the present time, nonsteroidal anti-inflammatory drugs (NSAIDs) were acids with similar pK_a values. On the other hand, we wondered why not all of them are inhibitors of prostaglandin synthesis (e.g., salicylic acid). Obviously, the physicochemical characteristics defining the pharmacokinetics of these compounds were important in controlling both the anti-inflammatory activity and the occurrence of typical side-effects. We shall not re-iterate the basic concepts of our hypothesis which is now widely acknowledged (Brune, 1974) but alluded to some recent refinements.

In 1974, we postulated, and still regard this to be true, that NSAIDs achieve particularly high concentrations in inflamed tissue, the wall of the small intestine and the stomach, the blood-stream, the liver, the kidney and the bone-marrow. Consequently, prostaglandin synthesis inhibition, as well as other effects in these target organs should contribute to both the anti-inflammatory and analgesic effects as well as tissue damage resulting in side-effects. Nevertheless, the clinical and, in part, experimental differences between the nonsteroidal drugs known at that time indicated that indeed differences in potency, and also distinct differences in the prevailance of side-effects may also be explained on the basis of the pharmacokinetic behaviour of these drugs which, in turn, would indicate ways and means to reduce these side-effects either by choosing the right drug for the right patient population or by further modifying the active structures towards compounds which have a good chance for better tolerability in patient populations at risk.

AVOIDING GASTRIC DAMAGE

Aspirin and other "classical" salicylates proved to be particularly damaging to the stomach. Later developments like diflunisal and more lipophilic acidic nonsteroidal drugs like diclofenac and ibuprofen were less toxic to the stomach (comp. e.g., Lanza, 1984). Moreover, stomach toxicity of aspirin could be reduced by acid-resistant coating of the drugs (McCormack and Brune, 1987). Acid resistant-coating, however, of diclofenac and other more lipophilic compounds did not reduce gastric toxicity. On the basis of these findings, we concluded that gastric absorption has the advantage of a fast and reliable onset of the therapeutic effects, it may, however, contribute to the incidence of the gastric side-effects. In a recent study, we could prove this hypothesis and show that gastric toxicity is less dependent on PG-synthesis but mainly dependent on the solubility of a NSAID at acidic pH and, by that, on the probable amount absorbed in the stomach (Fig. 1). We found a good correlation between these factors but still aspirin was even more gastrotoxic than expected from this relationship. Earlier results indicated that the acetyl moiety of aspirin is, in part, split-off during gastric absorption and transacetylation occurs which may add to the cytotoxic effects of salicylates in the stomach wall (Brune et al., 1979). The therapeutic consequence of the insight is that whenever fast onset of action is required and a NSAID (not a phenazone type or paracetamol type drug) is to be administered, gastric toxicity has to be taken into account. Whenever, however, slow onset of activitiy is possible, lipophilic compounds should be used, i.e. ibuprofen or diclofenac. Moreover, a reduced gastrotoxicity may also be achieved by prodrugs which do not encounter gastric absorption as, e.g., acemetacin or zwitter-

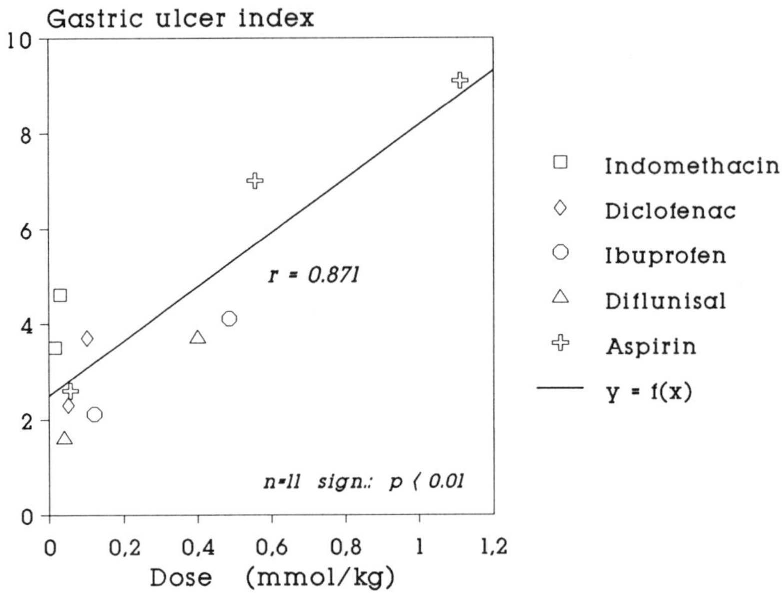

Fig. 1. Correlation between dose and gastric toxicity of NSAIDs in rats. NSAIDs were administered orally to fasted rats in two doses (aspirin in three doses). Gastric toxicity (ulcer index) strongly correlates with dose (mmol/kg body wt) given. Regression curve y = f(x). Doses per kg body wt p.o.: indomethacin 5 mg, 10 mg, diclofenac 15 mg, 30 mg, ibuprofen 25 mg, 100 mg, diflunisal 10 mg, 100 mg, aspirin 10 mg, 100 mg, 200 mg. (Beck et al., 1990a)

ions like azapropazone which, despite good hydrophilicity at acidic pH conditions, will not be absorbed in the stomach (McCormack and Brune, 1987). If the latter drugs are to be absorbed as fast as possible, salts may be administered on empty stomachs which might lead to fast transfer of the active ingredient towards the small intestine, i.e. facilitate absorption in the small intestine (Geisslinger et al., 1988). On the other hand, the additional acid-resistant coating of very lipophilic compounds, e.g., diclofenac, will not improve on the gastric toxicity, but may further retard absorption due to retention of the tablets or dragées in the stomach in some patients (Willis et al., 1979).

DECREASING INTESTINAL DAMAGE

Interestingly enough, prodrugs or very lipophilic drugs regularly show retarded absorption and reduced gastric toxicity, but may be harmful to the lower intestine. Moreover, the introduction of more lipophilic NSAIDs during the last thirty years has reduced the incidence of gastric ulcerations and perforations but, in parallel, there appears to be an increase in the incidence of duodenal, ileal and jejunal perforations (Walt et al., 1986). Moreover, early animal experiments show that the LD_{50} of, e.g., indomethacin in different species is defined by the occurrence of ileal and jejunal perforations but not by gastric damage (Duggan et. al., 1975). Moreover, it is obvious that the degree of hepatic elimination of a certain NSAID in a given species defines the LD_{50}. Finally, inflammation pharmacologists know that the LD_{50} of NSAIDs is generally low in dogs but relatively high, e.g., in monkeys correlating with the propensity of these drugs to be eliminated via bile (dog) or via kidney (monkey) (Duggan and Kwan, 1979). Finally, intestinal ulcerations occur in most species independent of the site of administration of the NSAID. These observations together with the apparent increase in ileal and jejunal toxicity of indomethacin when given in osmotic release forms (Del Favero, 1986) prompted us to postulate that the degree of enterohepatic circulation of the active ingredient defines the degree of intestinal toxicity of these compounds. Indeed, recent investigation in rats showed that the incidence and intensity of ileal and jejunal ulcerations was dependent on the degree of biliary excretion of unchanged drug or drug conjugated only (i.e. not the phase-I metabolites of the compound) and, in addition, on the potency of these compounds to block prostaglandin synthesis. Figure 2 summarizes our findings which may have some bearance on the clinical use of the NSAIDs and also on the development of additional compounds. Firstly, one may conclude that drugs with intensive enterohepatic circulation in man as indomethacin,

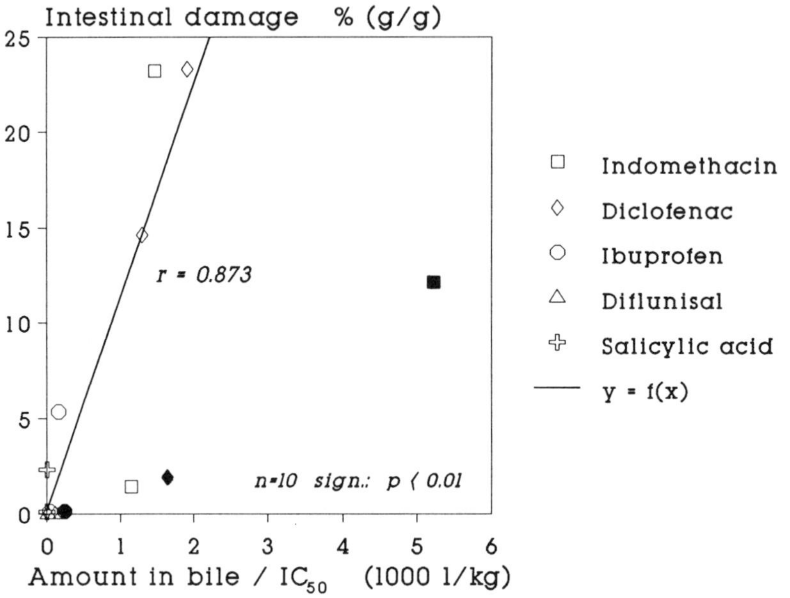

Fig. 2. Correlation between amount in bile/IC_{50} and intestinal toxicity of NSAIDs in rats. NSAIDs were administered orally (open symbols) to fed rats in two doses. Intestinal toxicity (% g/g of surface damaged) correlates with the amount of free and conjugated parent drug (µmol/kg body wt) excreted in bile divided by the cyclo-oxygenase inhibitory potency (IC_{50} value in mol/l) of the NSAIDs. Results obtained after intravenous treatment (closed symbols) are only shown but not included in the regression calculation. Regression curve y = f(x). Doses per kg body wt p.o.: indomethacin 5mg, 10 mg, diclofenac 15 mg, 30 mg, ibuprofen 25 mg, 100 mg, diflunisal 10 mg, 100 mg, aspirin 100 mg, 200 mg; doses per kg body wt i.v.: indomethacin 10 mg, diclofenac 30 mg, ibuprofen 100 mg (Beck et al., 1990a)

phenylbutazone and the oxicams should be avoided in risk groups, i.e. in elderly people, in which intensive enterohepatic circulation may go along with chronic impairment of either the blood-flow in the intestinal wall or atrophic changes of the intestinal mucosa. These drugs should be avoided, particularly if other compounds, which have less reliable therapeutic activity but also encounter less enterohepatic circulation, will suffice from clinical experience (Schneider et al., 1990). Moreover, ways and means to interfere with enterohepatic circulation of certain substances could be developed in order to amend their toxicity. It is presently under investigation if, for example, pharmacological and dietary means could do this job (Beck et al., 1990b). Finally, our findings explain the observation that for drugs with intensive enterohepatic circulation, parenteral or rectal administration may reduce the intestinal effects but will not prohibit them.

AVOIDING LIVER TOXICITY

It is well-known that all NSAIDs may cause gastrointestinal damage. It is less well-known that many of them may cause liver toxicity (Del Favero, 1988). In the past, many newly introduced NSAIDs were removed from the market-place due to liver toxicity (ibuphenac, sudoxicam, benoxaprofen). Diclofenac, which is probably the most widely-used NSAID world-wide, causes, with some regularity, an increase of liver derived transaminases (Kurowski, 1990). We have recently started looking for reasons for these effects. It occurred to us that intensive "first-pass" metabolisation of diclofenac is well-documented (Brune and Lanz, 1985). It may indicate that intensive hepatic metabolisation may cause the production of reactive intermediates which may then cause liver toxicity. Figure 3 gives some preliminary results. Indeed, diclofenac does enhance the toxicity of paracetamol in mice. This effect is, however, time-dependent, i.e. if diclofenac is given simultaneously with acetaminophen, it reduces the liver toxicity of paracetamol. If given before, it may enhance the toxicity. Further preliminary results indicate that diclofenac may be metabolised to reactive intermediates similiar to acetaminophen. These intermediates may cause toxicity either by direct effects or by exhausting the glutathione concentration of the liver. Of course, these preliminary results need further confirmation. They do,

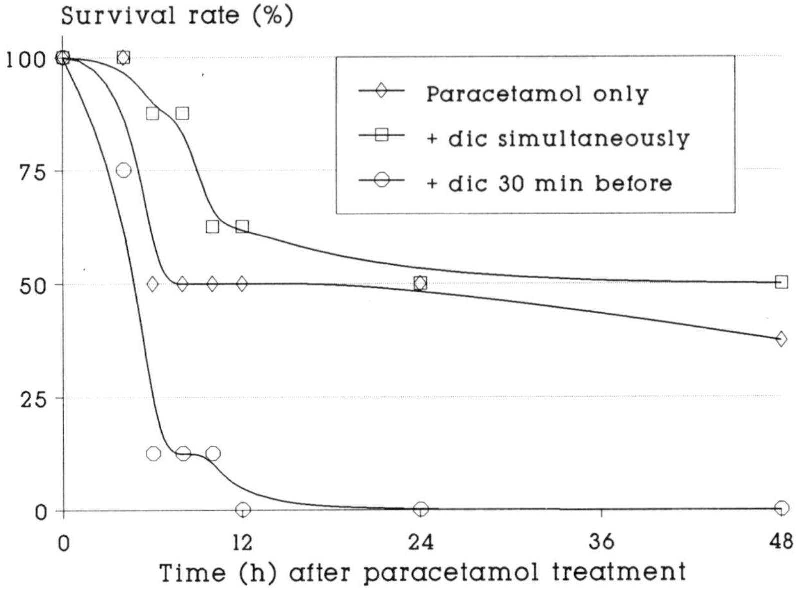

Fig. 3. Time course of survival rate of mice (% of n = 10), caused by paracetamol (600 mg/kg body wt intraperitoneal) given only and combined with diclofenac treatment (1 mg/kg body wt orally). Diclofenac was coadministered either 30 minutes before paracetamol or simultaneously. Abbreviation: dic = diclofenac

however, indicate ways and means to reduce the toxicity of diclofenac: Possibly diclofenac should be investigated as to which compounds could be given together with this NSAID, and those which should be avoided. Moreover, possibly supplementation with SH-group donors may reduce the toxicity of diclofenac.

THE PROBLEMS OF KIDNEY TOXICITY

Another site of the toxicity of NSAIDs is the kidney. As indicated earlier, a slow elimination of these drugs from the body which could be interpreted as the result of intensive intrarenal circulation, i.e. filtration in the glomerulus, secretion in the proximal tubulus and reabsorption in the distal tubulus, as indicated by earlier results (Lombardino, 1974), may cause functional disturbances of the renal function. On the other hand, potent NSAIDs with short elimination half-life as, e.g., suprophen, exerted acute morphological damage to the kidney (Del Favero, 1988). Again, it could be that intensive intrarenal circulation together with intensive inhibition of prostaglandin synthesis in the kidney cortex could blunt the blood perfusion of the papillae of the kidney, particularly in patients with hampered renal function. These reasonings are, however, so far pure speculations which need confirmation or rejection on the basis of experimental data. Only then, drugs with improved handling by the kidney and, thus, reduced kidney toxicity may be developed on a rational basis.

NEW TOOLS AND WAYS TOWARDS BETTER NSAIDS

Recently new possibilities for the development of more anti-inflammatory and more analgesic NSAIDs with less toxicity in one or the other organ systems have been developed. These are the pure enantiomers of 2-arylpropionic acids. Some of these enantiomers are transformed into each other within the living organism of man and animals (Williams, 1990). Others are not, and the pharmacokinetics of both enantiomers can be followed by enantioselective analytical methods (Menzel-Soglowek et al., 1990). Finally, the availability of the chemically pure enantiomer for animal experimentation and human investigation will allow for a re-evaluation of the contribution of prostaglandin synthesis inhibition for the activity of these drugs in terms of wanted and unwanted drug effects. First preliminary results indicate that enantiomers inhibiting prostaglandin synthesis are more potent in terms of anti-inflammatory action but also more damaging to the small intestine as compared to the non-prostaglandin synthesis inhibiting enantiomer. If so, the selective administration of either one enantiomer depending on the clinical condition would be feasible and advantageous. In other words, highly inflammatory processes should be treated by the enantiomer, which is a potent inhibitor of PG-synthesis, while less inflammation-related pain conditions would be the right indication for the alternative enantiomer.

REFERENCES

Beck, W.S., Schneider, H.T., Dietzel, K., Nuernberg, B., and Brune, K. (1990a) Gastrointestinal ulcerations induced by anti-inflammatory drugs in rats. Physicochemical and biochemical factors involved, Arch. Toxicol. 64, 210-217

Beck, W.S., Dietzel, K., Geisslinger, G., Engler, H., Vergin, H., and Brune K. (1990b) Effects of sodium salicylate on elimination kinetics of indomethacin and bile production in dogs, Drug Metab. Dispos. (in press)

Brune, K. (1974) How aspirin might work: a pharmacokinetic approach, Agents Action 4, 230-232

Brune, K. and Lanz, R. (1985) Pharmacokinetics of non-steroidal anti-inflammatory drugs. In: Handbook of inflammation, vol. 5: The Pharmacology of inflammation (I.L. Bonta, M.A. Bray, and M.J. Parnham, Eds), Elsevier Science Publishers, Amsterdam, New York, Oxford, pp. 413-449

Brune, K., Gubler H., and Schweitzer A. (1979) Autoradiographic methods for the evaluation of ulcerogenic effects of anti-inflammatory drugs, Pharmacol. Ther. 5, 199-207

Collier, H.O.J. (1984) The story of aspirin. In: Discoveries in pharmacology, vol. 2: Haemodynamics, hormones and inflammation (M.J. Parnham and J. Bruinvels, Eds), Elsevier Science Publishers, Amsterdam, New York, Oxford, pp. 555-593

Del Favero, A. (1986) Anti-inflammatory analgesics and drugs used in rheumatoid arthritis and gout. In: Side effects of drugs annual 10 (M.N.G. Dukes, Ed), Elsevier Science Publishers, Amsterdam, New York, Oxford, p. 76

Del Favero, A. (1988) Anti-inflammatory analgesics and drugs used in rheumatoid arthritis and gout. In: Side effects of drugs annual 12 (M.N.G. Dukes and L. Beeley, Eds), Elsevier Science Publishers, Amsterdam, New York, Oxford, p. 79

Dreser, H. (1907) Über modifizierte Salicylsäuren, Med. Klin. 3, 390-393

Duggan, D.E. and Kwan, K.C. (1979) Enterohepatic recirculation of drugs as a determination of therapeutic ratio, Drug Metab. Rev. 9, 21-41

Duggan, D.E., Hooke, K.F., Noll, R.M., and Kwan, K.C. (1975) Enterohepatic circulation of indomethacin and its role in intestinal irritation, Biochem. Pharmacol. 25, 1749-1754

Geisslinger, G., Dietzel, K., Bezler, H., Nuernberg, B., and Brune, K. (1988) Therapeutically relevant differences in the pharmacokinetical and pharmaceutical behaviour of ibuprofen lysinate as compared to ibuprofen acid, Int. J. Clin. Pharmacol. Ther. Toxicol. 27, 324-328

Kurowski, M. (1990) Das SPALA-Projekt. Erfassung unerwünschter Ereignisse unter der Therapie mit nichtsteroidalen Antirheumatika, Deutsche Apotheker Zeitung Nr. 16, 847-851

Lanza, F.L. (1984) Endoscopic studies of gastric and duodenal injury after the use of ibuprofen, aspirin, and other nonsteroidal anti-inflammatory agents, Am. J. Med. 77, 19-24

Lombardino, J.G. (1974) Enolic acids with anti-inflammatory activity. In: Medicinal chemistry. A series of monographs (G. deStevens, Ed): Anti-inflammatory agents. Chemistry and pharmacology, vol. 1 (R.A. Scherrer and M.W. Whitehouse, Eds), Academic Press, New York, San Francisco, London, pp. 129-157

McCormack, K. and Brune, K. (1987) Classical absorption theory and the development of gastric and mucosal damage associated with the nonsteroidal anti-inflammatory drugs. Arch. Toxicol. 60, 261-269

McCormack, K. and Brune, K. (1990) The amphiprotic character of azapropazone and its relevance to the gastric mucosa, Arch. Toxicol. 64, 1-6

Menzel-Soglowek, S., Geisslinger, G., and Brune, K. (1990) Stereoselective high-performance liquid chromatographic determination of ketoprofen, ibuprofen and fenoprofen in plasma using a chiral α_1 acid-glycoprotein column (enantiopac®), J. Chromatogr. (in press)

Rainsford, K.D. (1984) Aspirin and the salicylates, 1st ed., Butterworths, London, Boston, Durban, Singapore, Sidney, Toronto, Wellington

Rechenberg, H.K. v. (1957) Phenylbutazon - Butazolidin. Unter besonderer Berücksichtigung der Nebenwirkungen, G. Thieme Verlag, Stuttgart

Schneider, H.T., Nuernberg, B., Dietzel K., and Brune, K. (1990) Biliary elimination of non-steroidal anti-inflammatory drugs in patients, Br. J. Clin. Pharmacol. 29, 127-131

Walt, R., Katschinski, B., Logan, R., Ashley, J., and Langman, M. (1986) Rising frequency of ulcer perforation in elderly people in the United Kingdom, Lancet 1, 489-492

Williams, K.M. (1990) Enantiomers in arthritic disorders, Pharmacol. Ther. 46, 273-295

Willis, J.V., Kendall, M.J., Jack, D.B., Flinn, R.M., Thornhill, D.P., and Welling, P.G. (1979) The pharmacokinetics of diclofenac sodium following intravenous and oral administration, Eur. J. Clin. Pharmacol. 16, 405-410

AAS 32
Drugs in Inflammation

DEVELOPING NONSTEROIDAL ANTI-INFLAMMATORY DRUGS (NSAIDs) WITH DECREASED GASTROINTESTINAL (GI) TOXICITY

B. Goldlust, M. Doucette and C. Verduyn

Clinical Research, 3M Pharmaceuticals, St. Paul, MN, 55144, USA; and 3M Health Care Ltd, Loughborough, LE11 1EP, England

SUMMARY: NSAID-induced gastropathy is an important iatrogenic disorder that must be addressed in the development of NSAIDs. A scheme for clinical evaluation is described and salsalate is discussed as a prototype.

NSAID-induced gastropathy is now well-recognized (Roth & Bennett, 1987). The incidence of ulcers in chronic NSAID users is estimated to be 20% (eg., Gabriel & Bombardier, 1990). Perhaps 2-4000 deaths per year may occur in the US due to GI complications in rheumatoid patients who are chronic NSAID users (Fries, 1988).

The characteristics of NSAID gastropathy contrast with those of classic peptic ulcer disease (Roth & Bennett, 1987). For example, unlike classic peptic ulcer, NSAID-induced lesions are often asymptomatic. This underscores the substantial potential for morbid sequelae. The development of less GI-toxic NSAIDs is, therefore, an important objective.

CLINICAL EVALUATION

An NSAID developmental program to reduce GI toxicity may include prodrugs, formulation studies, or agents with different mechanisms of action (eg, non-prostaglandin inhibitors). Given appropriate preclinical testing, how does one go about determining clinically the potential for GI toxicity of an agent?

Since there is a poor correlation of GI complaints with mucosal injury in NSAID gastropathy, objective endpoints reflecting GI mucosal integrity are important. A scheme for clinical evaluation of GI toxicity potential is indicated in Table I. All the clinical models indicated have problems - methodologic or logistical, and are subject to interpretation. However, these models can be used to approach more optimal development of less GI-toxic drugs. After defining a safe dosage range, moderate to high dosages within that range are administered to normal healthy subjects to determine GI blood loss and effects on the hemostatic system, and to directly assess the short-term effects on the upper GI mucosa using endoscopy. Results of such endoscopic studies suggest a difference in the gastrotoxic potential among NSAIDs (Table II). Although all available data on NSAIDs are not included, an indication of relative GI mucosal toxicity is apparent. These data suggest that, at anti-inflammatory doses, all NSAIDs are not alike.

TABLE I. CLINICAL TESTING - GI TOXICITY

Phase I: Establish safe dosage range, then evaluate moderate to high dosages: - Cr^{51} - RBC - fecal blood loss - 2 wk. - Platelet function/bleeding time - $\leq$ 1 wk. - Normal subject endoscopy - 2 wk.	Phase III: Long-term ($\geq$1yr) GI tolerance studies(Pt) - Endoscopic - Hospitalization/ Bleeds
Phase II: Establish efficacious dosage range, then: - Endoscopic study in pts - 1-3 Mos	PhaseIV: - Postmarketing Surveillance

TABLE II. ENDOSCOPIC STUDIES OF NSAIDs IN SUBJECTS (Lanza, 1989)

Effect on Gastric Mucosa

Most Severe --> Least

Aspirin	Naproxen	Piroxicam	Salsalate
Buff. aspirin	Indomethacin	Enteric-aspirin	(Lanza et al, 1989)
Tolectin	Ibuprofen	Sulindac (also Graham et al, 1985)	

For examples, aspirin and tolectin are the most injurious and the non-acetylated salicylate, salsalate, the least injurious. This listing of NSAIDs represents a continuum of potential toxicity with some dose - toxicity relationships demonstrated. The predictability of long-term toxicity in these short-term studies (a few days to 2 weeks) requires further testing. However, these studies do provide preliminary indications of relative potential for GI toxicity. These short-term studies also provide a rational approach to differentiating chemical analogs, or determining priorities of development of two or more chemical series, as examples. After defining the efficacious dosage range, an endoscopic study in patients, eg elderly rheumatoids, should be considered (Table I). These studies should be at least 1-3 months in duration. Study design issues include stratification of entrants, eg prestudy NSAID, the need for a washout period, blinding, reference agent and dosages, and statistical power. Because of its high GI toxicity, plain aspirin is not a discriminating reference. If an agent continues to demonstrate a reduced potential for GI mucosal toxicity, then long-term studies (1 year or more) need to be considered. Endpoints may be ulcers (endoscopically) or hospitalizations for GI bleeds. Published long-term comparative endoscopic studies are rare or nonexistent and thus the reference NSAID to use is not clear. These studies are costly with large patient populations required, but they are needed. These and post-marketing surveillance studies are necessary to ascertain the relevance and predictability of shorter-term patient/subject endoscopic studies. Perhaps in the future, simpler, less expensive techniques to detect GI mucosal lesions will be available.

SALSALATE AS A PROTOTYPE

Anti-inflammatory doses of salsalate, a non-acetylated salicylate, show minimal deleterious effects in hemostatic and GI blood loss studies (Morris, et al., 1985; Ryan et al., 1986; Sweeney et al., 1988; Cohen, 1979). Endoscopic studies of up to 9 months' duration (Table III) have also been done in subjects or rheumatoid patients, utilizing therapeutic dosages of salsalate, naproxen, and piroxicam; or an analgesic dosage of enteric-coated aspirin. In every study, salsalate caused fewer and less serious GI mucosal lesions than the reference NSAID. Ulceration was observed with naproxen and piroxicam, but not with salsalate.

CONCLUSIONS

A plan for clinical evaluation of gastrotoxicity potential should be initiated early to optimize safety. Although the implications of endoscopic data are not fully understood, the relative risk of GI toxicity among NSAIDs delineated by such data should be considered in the development of new agents, as well as when initiating or substituting NSAID therapy in clinical practice. Clinical data suggest that salsalate has a relatively lower risk for GI mucosal toxicity.

TABLE III. ENDOSCOPIC STUDIES OF SALSALATE (SSA, 3-3.5 g/d)

Study	Design	Ref. Agent	Significant Findings
Scheiman et al., 1989	MD-Blind, Crossover-10 SS (6 Days)	Enteric-ASA (2.6 g/d)	Lesions: 6/10 (mod/sev) ASA 1/10 (mild) SSA
Lanza et al., 1989	MD-Blind, Parallel-40 SS (14 Days)	N (750 mg/d)	Lesions: 11/20 N 2/20 SSA
Bianchi Porro et al., 1989	Double-Blind, Parallel-39 Pts. (28 Days)	PIR (20 mg/d)	Ulcers: 5/20 PIR 0/19 SSA
Roth et al., 1990	MD-Blind, Parallel-39 Pts. (1-3 Mo;+6 Mo F/U)	N (750 mg/d; median)	Ulcers/erosions: 8/21 N 0/18 SSA

ASA = aspirin; N = naproxen; PIR = piroxicam; SS = subjects.

REFERENCES

Bianchi Porro, G., Petrillo, M., and Ardizzone, S. (1989). Salsalate in the treatment of rheumatoid arthritis: a double-blind clinical and gastroscopic trial versus piroxicam. II. Endoscopic evaluation. J. Int. Med. Res. 17, 320-323.

Cohen, A. (1979). Fecal blood loss and plasma salicylate study of salicylsalicylic acid and aspirin. J. Clin. Pharmacol. 19, 242-247.

Fries, J.F. (1988). Editorial. Postmarketing drug surveillance: Are our priorities right? J. Rheumatol. 15, 389-390.

Gabriel, S.E., and Bombardier, C. (1990). Editorial. NSAID induced ulcers. An emerging epidemic? J. Rheumatol. 17, 1-4.

Graham, D.Y., Smith, J.L., Holmes, G.I., and Davies, R.O. (1985). Nonsteroidal anti-inflammatory effect of sulindac sulfoxide and sulfide on gastric mucosa. Clin. Pharmacol. Ther. 38, 65-70.

Lanza, F.L. (1989). A review of gastric ulcer and gastroduodenal injury in normal volunteers receiving aspirin and other non-steroidal anti-inflammatory drugs. Scand. J. Gastroenterol. 24 (Suppl. 163), 24-31.

Lanza, F., Rack, M.F., Doucette, M., Ekholm, B., Goldlust, B., and Wilson, R. (1989). An endoscopic comparison of the gastroduodenal injury seen with salsalate and naproxen. J. Rheumatol. 16, 1570-1574.

Morris, H.G., Sherman, N.A., McQuain, C., Goldlust, M.B., Chang, S.F., and Harrison, L.I. (1985). Effects of salsalate (nonacetylated salicylate) and aspirin on serum prostaglandins in humans. Ther. Drug Monit. 7, 435-438.

Roth, S.H., and Bennett, R.E. (1987). Nonsteroidal anti-inflammatory drug gastropathy. Recognition and response. Arch. Intern. Med. 147, 2093-2100.

Roth, S., Bennett, R., Caldron, P., Hartman, R., Mitchell, C., Doucette, M., Ekholm, B., Goldlust, B., Lee, E., and Wilson, R. (1990). Reduced risk of NSAID gastropathy (GI mucosal toxicity) with nonacetylated salicylate (salsalate): an endoscopic study. Semin. Arthritis Rheum. 19 (Suppl. 2), 11-19.

Ryan, J., McMahon, F., Vargas, R., Gotzkowsky, S., McNamara, D., Kvam, D., Heide, M., and Ekholm, B. (1986). Effects of salsalate, aspirin and naproxen on plasma renin activity (PRA) and platelet thromboxane (T_xB_2) synthesis. Arthritis Rheum. 29 (Suppl. 4), S103.

Scheiman, J.M., Behler, E.M., Berardi, R.R., and Elta, G.H. (1989). Salicylsalicylic acid causes less gastroduodenal mucosal damage then enteric-coated aspirin. An endoscopic comparison. Dig. Dis. Sci. 34, 229-232.

Sweeney, J.D., Piedmont, M.P., Hoernig, L.A., and Fitzpatrick, J.F. (1988). The effect of salsalate on bleeding time, platelet aggregation in whole blood and the release reaction. Blood 72 (Suppl. 1), 311a.

AAS 32
Drugs in Inflammation

ANTI-INFLAMMATORY EFFICACY AND GASTROINTESTINAL IRRITANCY: COMPARATIVE 1 MONTH REPEAT ORAL DOSE STUDIES IN THE RAT WITH NABUMETONE, IBUPROFEN AND DICLOFENAC

R. Melarange, C. Gentry, C. O'Connell and P.R. Blower

SmithKline Beecham Pharmaceuticals, Coldharbour Road, Harlow, Essex, CM19 5AD, UK.

SUMMARY: Repeat oral dosing of nabumetone for 1 month maintains anti-inflammatory efficacy in a carrageenan model of paw oedema yet does not cause gastrointestinal damage. In contrast, ibuprofen or diclofenac, while also retaining anti-inflammatory activity, produced marked gastrointestinal irritancy as evidenced by mucosal damage and blood loss.

Nabumetone, a novel non-acidic drug, has been shown to be an effective anti-inflammatory drug in laboratory animals. Acute oral dosing studies in the rat demonstrated a better 'therapeutic' ratio (gastric irritancy: anti-inflammatory activity) compared with other non-steroidal anti-inflammatory drugs (Mangan, 1987). The present studies have involved extending the oral dosing period for 1 month to determine whether nabumetone's favourable acute dose profile was maintained compared with that of ibuprofen or diclofenac when given once daily in high anti-inflammatory doses.

MATERIALS AND METHODS

Drugs were orally administered once daily in 0.7% methyl cellulose to male Wistar rats (170-330g; n=6-10/group) using the following doses (5 x ID_{25} values obtained from previous carrageenan studies; mg/kg): nabumetone 79, ibuprofen 88 or diclofenac 11.5 respectively. The animals were weighed daily and their general health monitored closely. On day 27 they were fasted for 18h and on day 28 they received, 1h after drug treatment, a sub-plantar injection (0.1 ml) of 1% carrageenan into the right hind paw; 3h later paw oedema was measured plethysmographically. Animals were then killed and their stomachs removed and pinned onto cork boards. Damage, as evidenced by haemorrhagic petechia and ulcer, was assessed on a severity scale of 0-8 where 0-7 represented the degree of erosion formation and 8 the presence of one or more ulcers. Similarly, ulceration in the terminal ileum was assessed using a 0-8 scale were 0-6 represented the presence of ulcers, 7 for ulcers with nodules and adhesions and 8 for gut perforation. The caecum was dissected free and the contents removed and made up to 20 ml with distilled water and vortexed prior to centrifugation (400g for 10 min). Samples (0.5 ml) of the supernatant were then analysed for the presence of haemoglobin by a spectrophotometric assay as described previously (Clarke, 1971). Results were analysed using Student's 't' test or the Mann-Whitney 'U' test.

RESULTS

All three drugs produced significant inhibition ($p<0.05$-$p<0.001$) of carrageenan-induced paw oedema (Fig. 1).

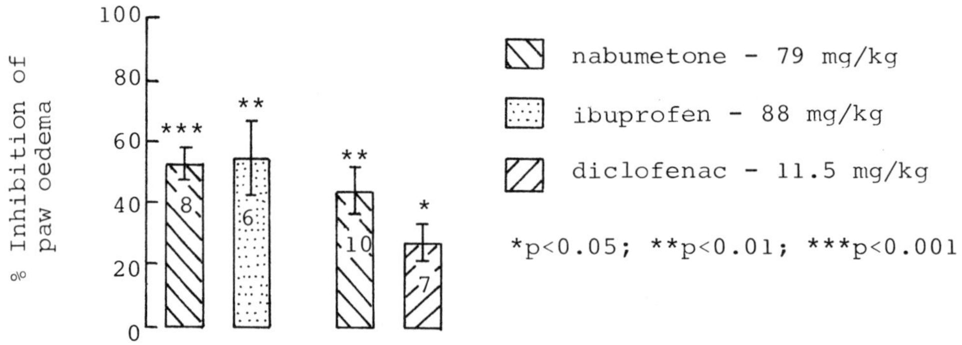

Figure 1. The effect of repeat dosing for 1 month of various NSAIDs on carrageenan paw oedema in the rat.

Gastric damage was induced by both ibuprofen and diclofenac and in some animals gastric ulcers were present. In contrast, nabumetone produced no gastric damage in either study (Fig. 2a). Ulcers, which were confined to the terminal ileum, were present in the ibuprofen and diclofenac groups but were absent in the nabumetone group where damage was not significantly greater compared with the control values (Fig. 2b).

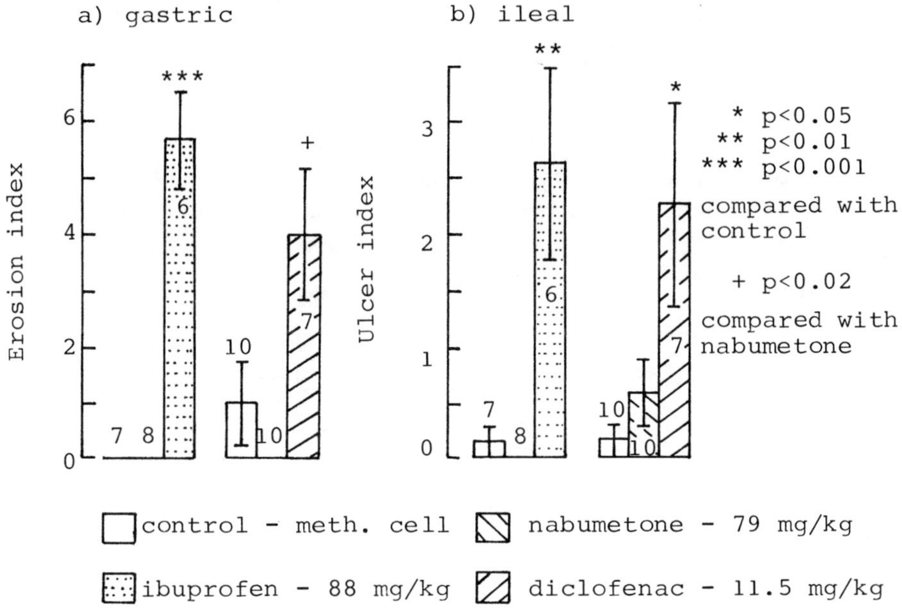

Figure 2. The effect of repeat dosing for 1 month of various NSAIDs on a) gastric and b) ileal damage in the rat.

In both studies, as a measure of gastrointestinal bleeding, caecal haemoglobin concentration was estimated. Fig. 3 shows that a small amount of haemoglobin was present in control animals which was not significantly altered by nabumetone. Ibuprofen increased the haemoglobin concentration above the control value by 268% ($p>0.05$) and diclofenac increased it by 52% ($p<0.05$).

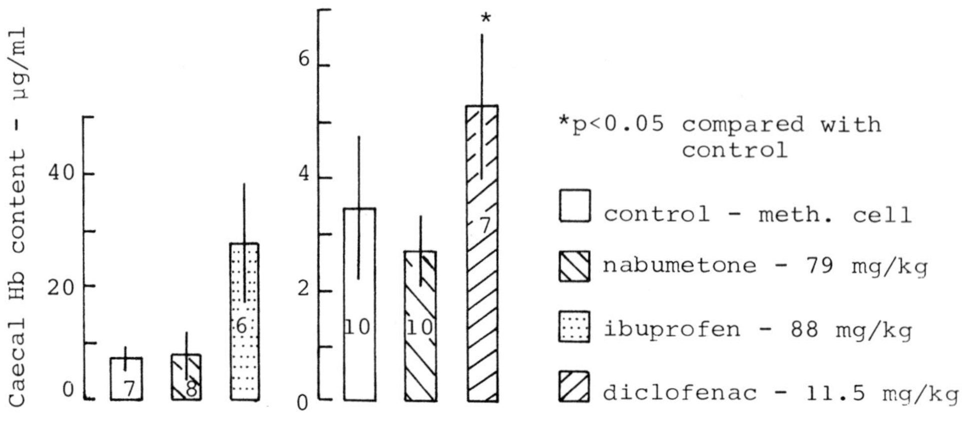

Figure 3. Caecal haemoglobin concentration (Hb) in rats after repeat oral dosing for 1 month with various NSAIDs

During the course of the studies, only diclofenac significantly reduced body weight gain compared with controls (days 3-20; $p<0.05-0.001$) and caused deaths (30%; Table I).

	$\bar{x}$ Body weight		Significance Level	% Mortality During Study
	Day 1	Day 20		
Control	320.8	393.7	-	0
nabumetone	329.8	392.5	NS	0
ibuprofen	326.0	388.4	NS	0
Control	170.5	315.7	-	0
nabumetone	169.0	306.2	NS	0
diclofenac	167.7	286.0	p<0.05	30

Table I. Changes in body weight during repeat dosing

DISCUSSION

In a previous study (Melarange et al, 1990) it was shown that nabumetone, when given acutely, produced effective inhibition of carrageenan paw oedema but failed to produce gastric damage. The results from the present study, where the oral dosing period was extended for 1 month, show that nabumetone maintains good anti-inflammatory activity yet does not cause gastrointestinal damage. Ibuprofen or diclofenac, however, while also retaining anti-inflammatory activity, produced marked gastrointestinal irritancy which was characterised by erosion and ulcer formation as well as blood loss. Nabumetone's favourable gastrointestinal profile may be partly attributable to its sparing effects on gastric mucosal prostanoid production (Melarange et al, 1990) and to the lack of biliary secretion of 6-methoxy-naphthyl acetic acid, the active metabolite (data on file).

CONCLUSION: Nabumetone, a non-acidic anti-inflammatory drug, when administered orally at a high anti-inflammatory dose for 1 month, was found to be well tolerated by the gastrointestinal mucosa. In contrast, ibuprofen or diclofenac in high anti-inflammatory doses induced gastrointestinal irritancy which was characterised by mucosal damage and bleeding.

REFERENCES

Clarke, B.S. (1971). A method for occult blood in faeces using non-carcinogenic reagents. Med. Lab. Tech., 28, 187-190.

Mangan, F.R. (1987). Nabumetone. In Non-Steroidal Anti-Inflammatory Drugs. A.J. Lewis and D.E. Furst, Eds, Marcel Dekker, New York, pp 439-472.

Melarange, R., Blower, P.R., Gentry, C. and O'Connell, C. (1990). Nabumetone, an effective anti-inflammatory agent, lacks the gastric irritancy potential of piroxicam or ibuprofen. Br. J. Pharmacol., 99, 172P.

AAS 32
Drugs in Inflammation

A NEW ANTIINFLAMMATORY AGENT (EGIS-5645) WITHOUT GASTROINTESTINAL SIDE-EFFECT

G. Gigler, E. Kiszelly, P. Tömpe, G. Kovács and K. Gadó

EGIS Pharmaceuticals, P.O.Box 100, H-1475 Budapest, Hungary

Summary: The compound EGIS-5645 is a potent antipyretic agent possessing analgesic and antiinflammatory properties. The drug is active in antiinflammatory models such as carrageenin oedema and adjuvant arthritis. EGIS-5645 shows practically no gastro-ulcerogenic effect. The molecule does not inhibit either prostaglandin biosynthesis or soybean lipoxygenase enzyme activity.

INTRODUCTION

EGIS-5645 (diaveridine: 2,4-diamino-5-[3,4-dimethoxy-benzyl]-pyrimidine), which inhibits folic acid metabolism, was applied against poultry coccidiosis (Jackson, 1966). In our animal experiments EGIS-5645 showed considerable antipyretic, analgesic and antiinflammatory activities. In contrast to the well known non steroidal antiinflammatory agents EGIS-5645 did not inhibit cyclooxygenase enzyme activity and did not produce gastrointestinal lesions even in an oral dose of 1000 mg/kg. The paper describes the main pharmacological properties of the compound.

MATERIALS AND METHODS

Antipyretic activity: A modification of the method of Fleming et al. (1969) was employed. The pyrexia of rats was induced by 2 ml of a 20 % aqueaous Brewer's yeast suspension injected s.c.

Carrageenin oedema: The method of Winter et al. (1962) was followed.

Adjuvant arthritis: The chronic inflammation was studied by the method of Newbould (1963) in male, Long Evans rats weighing 210-240 g.

Gastrointestinal toxicity: The acute experiment was performed according to the method of Wilhelmi and Menassé-Gdynia (1972). EGIS-5645 and indometacin were applied orally 6 and 16 h before the killing of animals by ether. The damages of gastric mucosa were registered in accordance with Adami et al. (1964). The 12-day study was carried out on the basis of the method of Schiantarelli and Cadel (1981). The test compounds were orally administered once a day for 12 consecutive days. The surviving rats were sacrified on the day after the final treatment and the small intestine was removed and the incidence rate of intestinal lesions was determined.

Influence on prostaglandin biosynthesis: Brain homogenates of Wistar rats were used as a source of cyclooxygenase enzyme. The prostaglandin synthesis was stimulated by noradrenaline. The homogenates (0.25 ml containing 0.05 M Tris-HCl buffer pH 7.4, and 0.15 M NaCl) were incubated with the test compounds and 10^{-3} M noradrenaline on 37 °C for 20 min. The reaction was terminated by placing the samples on ice bath. After centrifugation on 0 °C for 15 min, 1600 g, the PGF_{2alpha} content of the supernatant was determined by RIA (^3H-PGF_{2alpha} RIA kit was obtained from the Institute of Isotopes of the Hungarian Academy of Sciences).

Influence on lipoxygenase enzyme activity: The activity of the soybean 15-lipoxygenese enzyme (SERVA, 275,000 U/mg) was determined by the decreasing quantity of oxygene in the reaction mixture (10 ml) containing 0.1 M Borate buffer pH 9.0, 1 mg enzyme and the test compound. The reaction was initiated with 1 mg arachidonic acid (0.1 ml). Voltametric method was used to measure the decreasing levels of the oxygene with rotating platinum disc electrode (E_{RDE} = - 540 mV/Ag AgCl).

RESULTS

Table I gives a summary of the antipyretic and antiinflammatory activities of test compounds. The antipyretic effect of EGIS-5645 was comparable to the effect of aminophenazone and surpassed that of acetylsalicylic acid and paracetamol. The compound did not influence the body temperature of normothermic rats.

In the model of the rat hind paw oedema induced by carrageenin EGIS-5645 was more active than acetyilsalicylic acid, paracetamol, phenylbutazone, and less active than indometacin and piroxicam. In the adjuvant arthritis test in rats EGIS-5645 in an oral dose of 100 mg/kg proved to be as efficacious as 30 mg/kg phenylbutazone and 3 mg/kg indometacin and piroxicam.

Table I: Antipyretic and antiinflammatory activities of EGIS-5645 and the reference compound in rats.

Compound	Dose mg/kg p.o.	Antipyreyic activity at 3 h after treatment ΔT (°C)	% inhibition in carrageenin oedema test
EGIS-5645	100	- 1.61**	51.2**
	200	- 2.48**	48.4**
Acetylsalicylic	100	- 1.13*	34.1**
acid	200	- 1.03*	44.2**
Paracetamol	100	- 1.34*	16.2
	200	- 1.38**	30.1**
Aminophenazone	100	- 1.70**	nt
	200	- 2.23**	nt
Phenylbutazone	100	nt	55.8**
	200	nt	55.8**
Indometacin	5	nt	43.0*
	10	nt	56.3**
Piroxicam	5	nt	57.7**
	10	nt	67.0**

Significance of differences from controls (* $p<0.05$, ** $p<0.01$) were calculated by Duncan's test (antipyretic activity) and Student's t-test (antiinflammatory activity); nt not tested.

In acute gastrointestinal toxicity experiment indometacin increased the ulcus frequency and ulcus index depending on the dose, EGIS-5645 induced only small alteration even in high doses (1000 mg/kg), this effect of the compound was independent of the dose employed. Table II gives the mortality caused by intestinal perforation following repeated daily oral treatment. Although after the highest dose of EGIS-5645 a high incidence of mortality could be observed in the rats, this was definitely not caused by intestinal perforation. In contrast to the doses of indometacin and piroxicam after which the cause of mortality was mostly intestinal perforation. As far as the small intestine was concerned no ulcus was developed when using EGIS-5645, whereas the reference compounds bought about its occurence.

Table II: Intestinal perforation in the rat after 12-day oral administration of EGIS-5645 and the reference compounds.

Compound	Daily dose mg/kg p.o.	Dead/ treated animals	Frequency of lethal intestinal perforation	Frequency of ulcus in small intestine
Control	-	0/10	0/10	0/10
EGIS-5645	500	0/10	0/10	0/10
	1000	6/10	0/10	0/10
Indometacin	4	1/10	1/10	1/ 9+
	8	9/10	8/10	4/ 6+
Piroxicam	20	0/10	0/10	0/10
	40	3/10	3/10	2/ 9+

+ Data of rats died during the night were omitted.

EGIS-5645 (10^{-8}-10^{-3} M) did not hinder the noradrenaline stimulated release of prostaglandin from rat brain homogenate, while indometacin (IC_{50} = 2.1 10^{-6} M), piroxicam (IC_{50} = 1.7 10^{-5} M) and phenylbutazone (IC_{50} = 1.9 10^{-4} M) inhibited PGF_{2alpha} release. EGIS-5645 (10^{-7}-10^{-5} M) was inactive against 15-lipoxygenase enzyme from soybean, while NDGA (IC_{50} = 1.0 10^{-6} M) and phenidone (IC_{50} = 7.0 10^{-7} M) were potent in inhibiting of enzyme activity.

DISCUSSION

The compound EGIS-5645 was as potent as aminophenazone considering the antipyretic property. The drug showed significant analgesic effect in acetic acid induced writhing test and in Randall-Selitto model in rats (Gigler et al., 1988). The molecule exerted inhibitory activity in carrageenin induced rat paw oedema and also in adjuvant arthritis assays.

Both after single and repeated oral administration EGIS-5645 did not induce ulceration of the gastrointestinal mucosa. In contrast to the NSAIDs EGIS-5645 did not inhibit the biosynthesis of prostaglandins or soybean 15-lipoxygenase.

EGIS-5645 blocked the luminol induced chemiluminescence of human leukocytes, indicating an antioxidant property without scavanger activity. Its effect surpassed that of the reference antiinflammatory agents by several order of magnitude (Gigler et al., 1988). The acute toxicity of EGIS-5645 was much more favourable than that of the classical NSAIDs. Although the mode of action of EGIS-5645 has not been clear yet, its strong antioxidant property may explain the effects of this compound.

REFERENCES

Adami, E., Marazzi-Ubertti, E., and Turba, C. (1964): Pharmacological Research on Gefarnate, a New Synthetic Isoprenoid with an Anti-Ulcer Action, Arch. Int. Pharmacodyn. 147, 113-145.

Fleming, J.S., Bierwagen, M.E., Pircio, A.W., and Pindell, M.H. (1969): A New Anti-Inflammatory Agent 1-(4-Clorobenzoyl)-3-(5-Tetrazolylmethyl)-Indole (BL-R743), Arch. Int. Pharmacodyn. 178, 423-433.

Gigler, G., Petőcz, L., Gadó, K., Kiszelly, E., and Fekete, M.I.K. (1988): The Pharmacology of a New Antiinflammatory Agent EGIS-5645, Pharm. Res. Comm. 20, Suppl. I. 191-192.

Jackson, N. (1966): A Comparison of the Toxicity of the Coccidiostats Diaveridine and Pyrimethamine in the Chick and the Effect of an Antibiotic on the Anti-Folic Activity of Pyrimethamine, Res. vet. Sci. 7, 196-206.

Newbould, B.B. (1963): Chemotherapy of Arthritis Induced in Rats by Mycobacterial Adjuvant, Brit. J. Pharmacol. 21,127-136.

Schiantarelli, P., and Cadel, S. (1981): Piroxicam Pharmacologic Activity and Gastrointestinal Damage by Oral and Rectal Route, Arzneim.-Forsch./Drug. Res. 31(I), 87-92.

Wilhelmi, G., amd Menassé-Gdynia, R. (1972): Gastric Mucosal Damage Induced by Non-Steroid Anti-Inflammatory Agents in Rats of Different Ages, Pharmacology 8, 321-328.

Winter, C.A., Risley, E.A., and Nuss, G.W. (1962): Carrageenin-Induced Edema in Hind Paw of the Rat as an Assay for Antiinflammatory Drugs, Proc. Soc. Exp. Biol. Med. 111, 544-547.

AAS 32
Drugs in Inflammation

ANTIPYRETIC ACTIVITY OF TEBUFELONE (NE-11740) IN MAN

J.H. Powell, and M.P. Meredith
The Procter & Gamble Co., Miami Valley Laboratories Cincinnati, Ohio, USA

R. Vargas, F.G. McMahon, and A.K. Jain
Clinical Research Center, New Orleans, Louisiana, USA

ABSTRACT

Tebufelone (formerly NE-11740) is a member of the new class of *di-tert-butyl-phenol* anti-inflammatory agents. It has previously been reported that this new agent has potent analgesic, antipyretic, and anti-inflammatory effects using *in vitro, in vivo,* and *ex vivo* experimental models. A randomized, active- and placebo- controlled double-blinded study in 120 healthy males, 20 to 55 years old, was conducted to clinically assess tebufelone's antipyretic activity. Subjects received a single peroral dose of placebo, 650 mg aspirin (ASA), or tebufelone at doses of 25, 50, 100, or 200 mg. Thirty minutes later, *E. coli* endotoxin (2 ng/kg) was administered intravenously. Oral temperatures were recorded at 15 minute intervals from 30 minutes post dosing to 8 hours post endotoxin administration. Areas under the temperature curves (AUCs), adjusted for baseline, were significantly lower than placebo for ASA and all but the 25 mg tebufelone groups. An AUC dose-response equation estimates 60 mg tebufelone as equivalent to 650 mg ASA, with 50 mg tebufelone not significantly greater than 650 mg ASA. Side effects, attributable to the endotoxin, included mild flu-like symptoms and were worse in the placebo group and the non-efficacious 25 mg tebufelone group. Doses of 100 and 200 mg tebufelone had onset characteristics indistinguishable from 650 mg ASA, whereas 50 mg tebufelone showed significantly slower onset while suppressing temperature for a longer period than ASA. These results provide an important early demonstration of tebufelone's biological activity in man.

OBJECTIVES OF STUDY

Quantify the antipyretic effects and dose-response of a single peroral dose of tebufelone (25, 50, 100, and 200 mg) compared with placebo and 650 mg ASA.

Specifically:

- Characterize tebufelone's dose-response for area under the temperature progress curve (AUC)

- Estimate tebufelone dose that gives an AUC equivalent to 650 mg ASA
- Characterize the onset behavior of tebufelone versus placebo and ASA
- Examine the rate of temperature change across time for tebufelone versus placebo and 650 mg ASA
- Examine frequency of commonly reported complaints due to the endotoxin

MATERIALS & METHODS

A total of 120 healthy male volunteers participated in this study. Subjects passing usual clinical screening criteria were admitted to the ward on the evening prior to the designated study day. They were housed in a comfortable room with a controlled temperature of 70°F.

Baseline oral temperatures were taken 3 times, 15 minutes apart, using an electronic thermometer (IVAC model 2000). Subjects continued on the study if their temperature was between 97.4 and 98.8°F, and if their highest and lowest values differed by no more than 0.2°F.

Subjects meeting the inclusion criteria were randomly allocated to 6 groups of 20. Each group received a single peroral dose of either tebufelone at 25, 50, 100, or 200 mg, or placebo, or 650 mg ASA. After 30 minutes they received 2 ng/kg *E. coli* endotoxin intravenously. Oral temperatures and complaints were elicited every 15 minutes for 8 hours.

DEMOGRAPHIC DATA FROM STUDY POPULATION

Group	Age (yr)	Weight (kg)	Height (cm)	Race	
				Black	Caucasian
Placebo	36 ± 9[†]	71.1 ± 8.6	175 ± 5	7	13
Tebufelone					
25 mg	34 ± 9	74.5 ± 8.8	175 ± 7	5	15
50 mg	35 ± 11	77.4 ± 14.6	176 ± 10	7	13
100 mg	36 ± 10	78.7 ± 12.2	180 ± 8	10	10
200 mg	36 ± 10	70.1 ± 10.9	177 ± 9	7	13
650 mg ASA	35 ± 9	71.0 ± 10.8	175 ± 6	6	14

[†] Mean ± Standard deviation

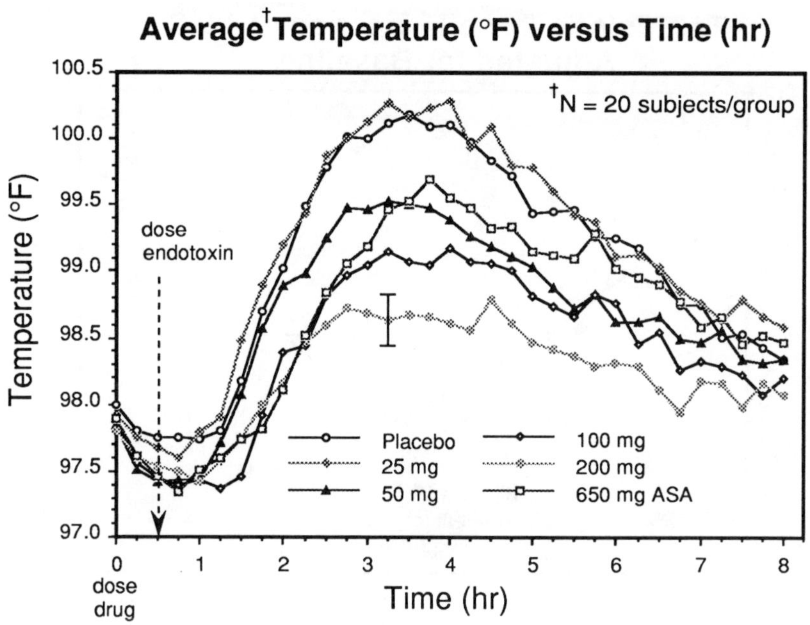
Average[†] Temperature (°F) versus Time (hr)
[†]N = 20 subjects/group
Temperature (°F)
dose endotoxin
dose drug
Time (hr)
Placebo
25 mg
50 mg
100 mg
200 mg
650 mg ASA

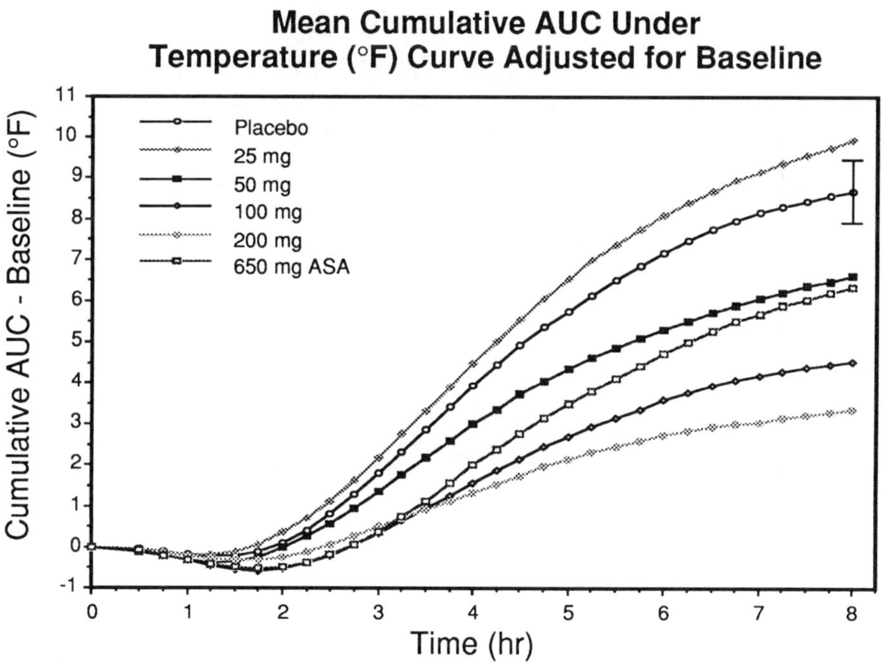
Mean Cumulative AUC Under Temperature (°F) Curve Adjusted for Baseline
Cumulative AUC - Baseline (°F)
Time (hr)
Placebo
25 mg
50 mg
100 mg
200 mg
650 mg ASA

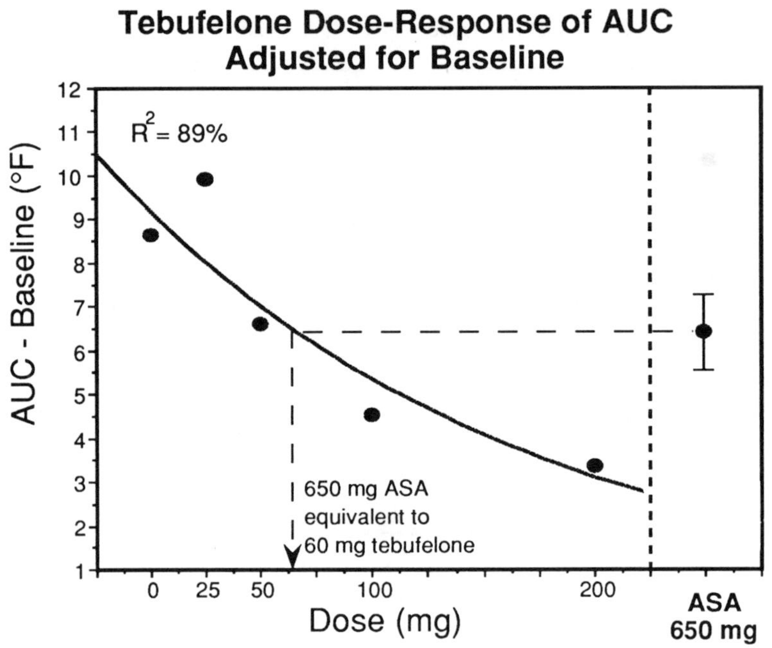

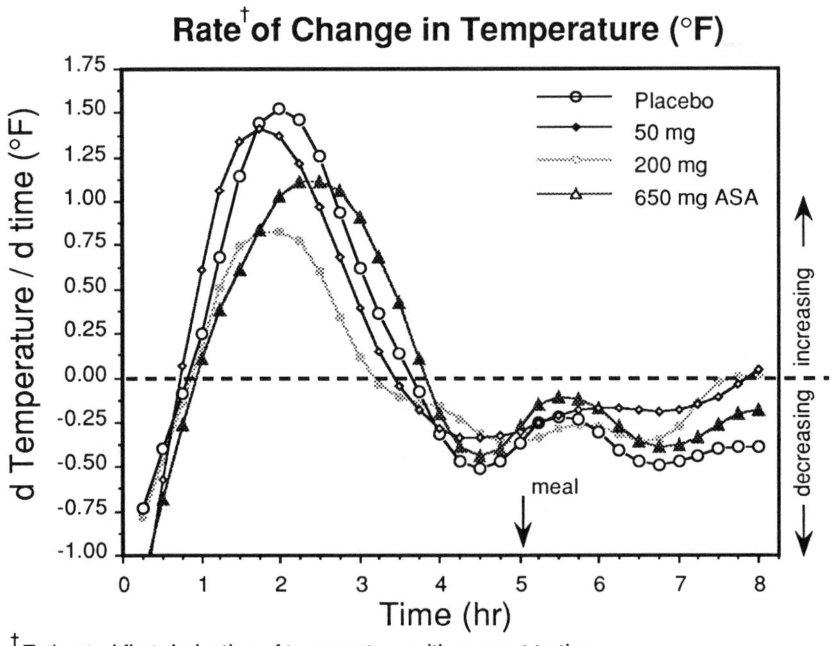

†Estimated first derivative of temperature with respect to time

FREQUENCY OF MOST OFTEN REPORTED COMPLAINTS

Group	Myalgia	Chills	Headache	None
Placebo	12	13	15	2
Tebufelone				
25 mg	14	17	13	2
50 mg	9	9	10	3
100 mg	10	8	10	7
200 mg	6	5	8	7
650 mg ASA	9	8	9	4

CONCLUSIONS

- Tebufelone is biologically active in man and further clinical development should proceed
- Significant tebufelone dose-response for temperature AUC was demonstrated
- 60 mg tebufelone has equivalent antipyretic activity to 650 mg ASA
- 200 mg tebufelone demonstrated a significantly lower AUC than 650 mg ASA over the 8 hours of study
- 100 and 200 mg tebufelone had antipyretic onset rates indistinguishable from 650 mg ASA
- Frequency of complaints decreased with increasing tebufelone dose
- Rates of temperature decrease were significantly faster for 200 mg tebufelone than for 650 mg ASA over the first 4 hours

ACKNOWLEDGEMENTS

We would like to thank J.E. Brooks, E.C. Drago, and J.V. Damo of Procter & Gamble's Miami Valley Laboratories for assistance in preparing this poster for presentation. K.R. Hicks was responsible for producing the final protocol and monitoring the execution of this study.

STEROID-SAVING POTENCY OF NONSTEROIDAL ANTIINFLAMMATORY AGENTS - A REEVALUATION WITH THE NEW AGENT CGP 28238 IN RAT INFLAMMATORY MODELS

R. Hirschelmann, [1]G. Pöch, Ines Rafler, O. Rickinger, and J. Giessler

Lehrstuhl für Pharmakologie, Sektion Pharmazie, Martin-Luther-Universität Halle-Wittenberg, Halle (Saale), DDR-4010 and [1]Institut für Pharmakodynamik und Toxikologie, Graz, A-8010

SUMMARY: The steroid-saving activity of the highly potent new non-steroid antiinflammatory agent CGP 28238 was determined in rat carrageenin paw edema and in primary phase of adjuvant arthritis in comparison with indomethacin. Both nonsteroidal agents showed independent synergistic effects with dexamethasone. Thereby, both compounds reduced the dose of the glucocorticoid necessary for equieffective inhibition of inflammation in the same dose range.

Steroidal anti-inflammatory agents are able to suppress the severest inflammatory reactions in rheumatoid arthritis and ther immunological diseases. However, these beneficial actions are inevitably associated with life-threatening side effects. Therefore, the nonsteroidal antiinflammatory agents are used in combination with glucocorticoids for reducing the doses of steroids which consequently diminishes their dangerous side effects (Mathies, 1973). Since the mode of action of steroids and nonsteroids is evidently different, their combination may correspond to, or even exceed, independent interactions; the latter would indicate true potentiating antiinflammatory effects, in view of the possible mode of action of the two substance classes: a sequential inhibition of arachidonic acid metabolism. The potent new nonsteroidal antiinflammatory agent CGP 28238 (6-(2,4-difluorophenoxy)-5-methylsulfonylamino-1-indanone) does not inhibit PG-synthase in sheep seminal vesicle (SSV) microsomal preparations, contrary to the aspirin-like nonsteroids, although CGP 28238 is a potent inhibitor of PG synthesis in cellular systems (Wiesenberg et al., 1989). We have found that CGP 28238 even antagonizes cyclooxygenase inhibition of aspirin or indomethacin in SSV preparations (Hirschelmann et al., 1990). Thus, its role in arachidonic acid metabolism in vivo during inflammation remains to be established.

In the present case we deal with the interaction of CGP 28238 with the glucocorticoid dexamethasone in rat inflammatory models in comparison to the PG-synthase inhibitor indomethacin.

MATERIAL AND METHODS

Female rats of an outbread Wistar strain (WIST: BARBY), b. w. 100-160 g, starved for 20-24 hours, but they had free access to drinking water. Carrageenin paw edema and primary adjuvant inflammation (adjuvant edema) were induced as described elsewhere (Hirschelmann and Bekemeier, 1979).

Substances used: CGP 28238 (CIBA-GEIGY AG, Basel); dexamethasone (Organon, OSS); indomethacin (Merck Sharp & Dohme, Rahway).

Calculation of independent effects: Independent effects were estimated at the indicated time points in Fig. 1 on the basis of the assumption that a drug A in the presence of a drug B, independently interacting with drug A, causes the same reduction of the edema as in the absence of drug B. Briefly, the reduction by drug A to a fraction of the control value was first determined. Then, the same reduction from the value observed in the presence of drug B was estimated, which corresponds to the expected value of independent interaction.

Statistics: The time-course values of combined effects observed in individual experiments were compared with the expected values. The number of experiments observed below (or above, respectively) the expected median values were compared with N/2 (Pöch et al., 1990); $p < 0.05$ was taken to indicate significant differences between observed and expected effects.

RESULTS

As shown in Fig.1a,b, the combination of CGP 28238 with dexamethasone caused independent interactions in primary adjuvant inflammation and in carrageenin edema, as well. Comparable results were obtained with indomethacin (Fig. 1c). Thus, the time-effect curves show no essential differences in the independent synergistic interaction between CGP 28238 and indomethacine when combining these agents with dexamethasone. Combination treatment caused effects which apparently allow to safe about 50 % of the glucocorticoid dose (Table I). In contrast, combination of the two nonsteroidal antiinflammatory agents with each other apparently resulted in antagonism (Fig. 1d; Table I).

DISCUSSION

The results of the present experiments show independent interactions between the nonsteroidal antiinflammatory agent CGP 28238 and dexamethasone with respect to inhibition of edema, resembling the interaction between indomethacin and the glucocorticoid. Had the combined effects exceeded the effects of independently interacting compounds, it would have supported a sequential inhibition of the arachidonic acid metabolism as the (main) mechanism responsible for the observed interaction. Also, in previous observations (Bekemeier and Hirschelmann, 1986) no statistically significant evidence for a sequential type of combined action between cyclooxygenase-inhibitors as nonsteroidal antiinflammatory agents and dexamethasone was obtained in carrageenin edema and adjuvant arthritis.

Theoretically, one could also argue that the observed combined effect is the resultant of two opposing actions. Then, a marked synergistic interaction due to sequential interaction in the arachidonic metabolism could have been weakened, or even reversed, by an antagonistic component in the interaction. Furthermore, antagonism could occur when the synergistic component is less pronounced. As a matter of fact, van Arman et al. (1973) have reported on antagonism between antiinflammatory agents. These authors found an antagonism between the nonsteroids, aspirin and indomethacin, in rat adjuvant arthritis, a result which is in line with our data with the CGP/indomethacin combination. They also reported on antagonism between the steroids, hydrocortisone and prednisolone, on the one hand and aspirin on the other hand.

It is not clear whether the antagonistic effect of CGP 28238 against indomethacin-induced inhibition of PG-synthase in vitro (Hirschelmann et al., 1990; the pA_2 value was found to be ca. 4.3) is the mechanism by which this compound antagonizes the antiinflammatory effect of indomethacin in vivo. Irrespective of the precise mechanism(s) of interactions, our results show that CGP 28238, like indomethacin, possesses a steroid-saving effect. The combination of CGP 28238 reduced the dose of dexamethasone to about one half without loss of the antiinflammatory effect in rats. From the results with experimental inflammation, a similar effect of CGP 28238 can be anticipated in human inflammatory disorders.

Table I: Inhibition of primary adjuvant inflammation. The substances were administered from day 1 until day 4, once daily. n=8 per group.

Experiment No.	Substance mg/kg p.o.	Inhibition (%) 2d	3d	4d	5d
I	Dexameth. 0.1	45	56	58	61
II	Dexameth. 0.05	23	30	42	53
	CGP 28238 2.0	10	30	36	37
	Dex. + CGP 0.05 + 2.0	38	58^{+}	69^{+}	70^{+}
III	Dexameth. 0.025	10	27	35	25
	CGP 28238 1.0	9	34	42	45
	Indom. 1.0	10	23	32	25
	Dex. + CGP 0.025 + 1.0	39^{+}	49^{+}	60^{+}	54^{+}
	Dex. + Indom. 0.025 + 1.0	41^{+}	55^{+}	53^{+}	46^{+}
IV	CGP 28238 2.0	14	36	51	55
	Indom. 0.5	10	43	49	52
	CGP + Indom. 2.0 + 0.5	13	22^{++}	37^{++}	45

$^{+}$ Significantly different ($p < 0.05$; Student's t-test) from the respective dexamethasone group. $^{++}$ Significantly different ($p < 0.05$; Student's t-test) from the respective monotherapy group.

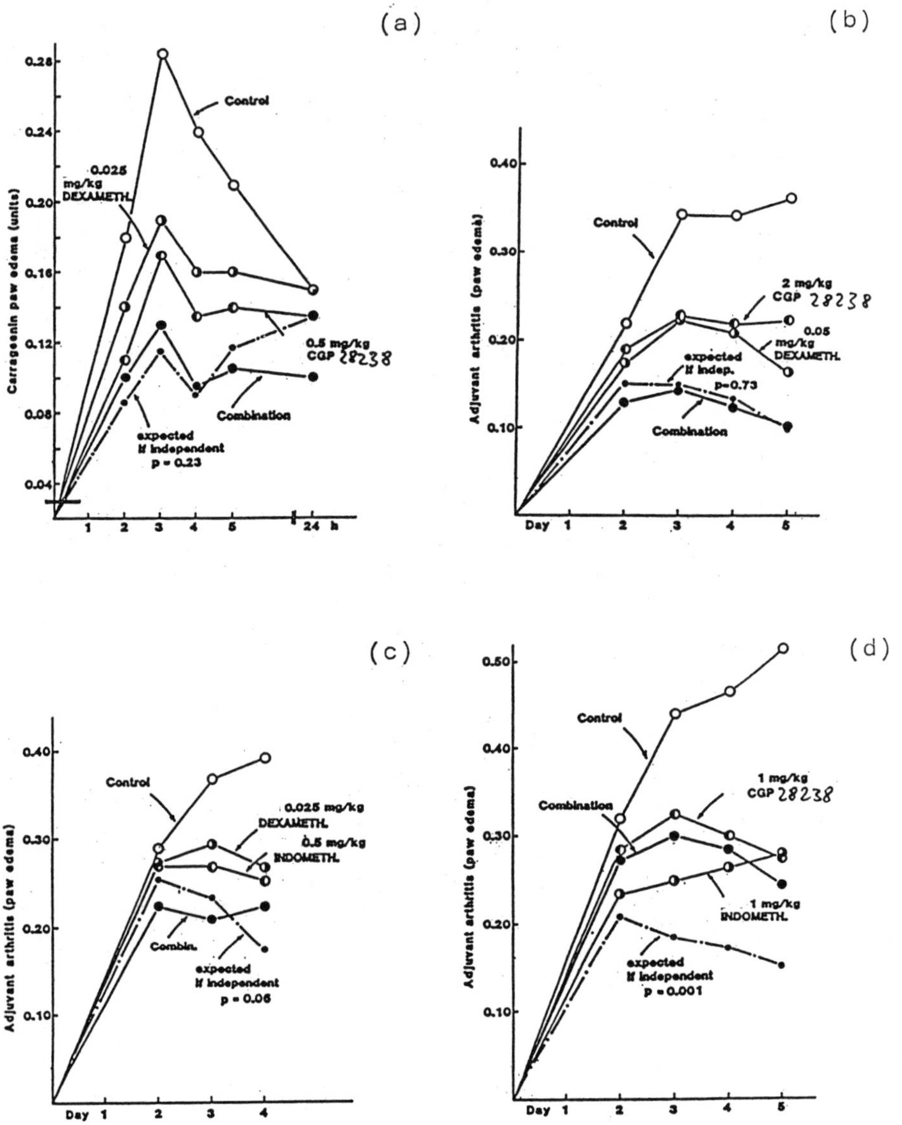

Fig. 1.

Development of carrageenin paw edema (panel a) and of primary adjuvant inflammation (panel b) after dexamethasone/CGP combination as well as of adjuvant inflammation after indomethacin/dexamethasone treatment (panel c). Panel d: Adjuvant inflammation after CGP/indomethacin treatment. Median values of 6 to 8 animals.

REFERENCES

van Arman, C. G., Nuss, G. W., and Risley, E. A. (1973), Interactions of Aspirin, Indomethacin and other Drugs in Adjuvant-Induced Arthritis in the Rat, J. Pharmacol. Exp. Therap. 187, 400-414.

Bekemeier, H., and Hirschelmann, R. (1986), On Steroid-saving Drug Combinations in Carrageenin Edema and Adjuvant Arthritis, Arzneim.-Forsch./Drug Res. 36, 1521-1524.

Hirschelmann, R., and Bekemeier, H. (1979), On the role of peroxidase and catalase reactions in inflammation, Int. J. Tiss. Reac. I, 11-20.

Hirschelmann, R., Hentschel, M., and Gießler, J. (1990), CGP 28238, a new nonsteroidal antiinflammatory agent: Relation to arachidonic acid metabolism, Abstract P3, 12th European Workshop on Inflammation, Halle (Saale), 3o-31 May.

Mathies, H. (1973), Aktuelle Steroidprobleme. Dr. Dietrich Steinkopff Verlag, Darmstadt.

Pöch, G., Dittrich, P., and Holzmann, S. (1990), Evaluation of combined effects in dose-response studies by statistical comparison with additive and independent interactions, J. Pharmacol. Methods, in press.

Pöch, G., Dittrich, P., and Holzmann, S. (1990), Evaluation of combined effects in dose-response studies with the aid of "ALLFIT" and the χ^2 goodness-of-fit statistic, Naunyn-Schmiedeberg's Arch. Pharmacol. Suppl. to Vol. 341, R 1 (1990).

Wiesenberg-Böttcher, I., Schweizer, A., Green, J. R., Seltenmeyer, Y., and Müller, K. (1989), The pharmacological profile of CGP 28238, a highly potent anti-inflammatory compound, Agents and Actions 26, 240-242.

AAS 32
Drugs in Inflammation

A BIOCHEMICAL INVESTIGATION OF AURANOFIN NEPHROTOXICITY BY HIGH FIELD PROTON NUCLEAR MAGNETIC RESONANCE (NMR) SPECTROSCOPY

Martin GROOTVELD*, Andrew W.D. CLAXSON, Declan NAUGHTON and David R. BLAKE

Inflammation Group, The London Hospital Medical College, London, E1 2AD, U.K.

*Author to whom correspondence should be addressed

SUMMARY

High-field proton NMR spectroscopic analysis of urine and plasma has been employed to study the biochemical effects and nephrotoxic action of an intramuscular dose of auranofin in rats. Auranofin induced a characteristic profile of proximal tubular damage as evidenced by aminoaciduria, lactic aciduria and increased urinary acetate concentrations. In addition, ethanol was detectable in both urine and plasma obtained from auranofin-treated rats.

Auranofin-mediated elevations in the plasma and urine concentrations of 3-D-hydroxybutyrate indicated an increased utilisation of fats for fuel in rats treated with this novel therapeutic agent.

INTRODUCTION

The highly lipophilic, orally-active ternary two-coordinate gold(I) complex auranofin (2,3,4,6-tetra-0-acetyl-1-thio-ß-D-glucopyranosato-S-(triethylphosphine) gold(I)) has been shown to be an effective second-line therapeutic agent for the treatment of inflammatory joint diseases (Sutton, B.M. (1983)). However, the renal complications of therapy with gold(I) complexes are well known (Freyberg, R.H. (1966)). Although Markiewicz et al (1988) have described the ability of auranofin to produce a species-specific heavy metal nephrotoxicity in animals, little is known about the induction and consequences of these nephrotoxic lesions at the molecular level.

In order to investigate the ability of auranofin to influence biochemical parameters *in vivo*, and, on a more general level, its cumulative toxicological properties or those associated with high dosage levels, we have employed high field proton Hahn spin-echo NMR spectroscopy to assess the metabolic status of urine and blood plasma obtained from animals treated with this novel therapeutic agent.

MATERIALS AND METHODS

Animals and treatment A group of male Wistar albino rats (n = 6) were treated with auranofin which was administered intramuscularly as a suspension in 0.9% (w/v) NaCl to give a dose level of 99 mg/kg. Throughout the experiment, food and tap water were allowed *ad libitum*. Urine was collected immediately before and at 12 and 24 hr. after dosing. Plasma was sampled immediately before and at 1, 12 and 24 hr. post dosing.

NMR measurements Proton NMR measurements were carried out on a Bruker WH 400 spectrometer operating in quadrature detection mode at 400 MHz. All spectra were recorded at a probe temperature of 25°C. Typically, 0.55 ml of a urine or plasma sample was placed in a 5 mm diameter NMR tube, and 0.06 ml of D_2O was added to provide a field-frequency lock. The broad protein resonances and the intense water signal were suppressed by a combination of the Hahn spin-echo sequence (90°-τ- 180°-τ-collect; τ = 60 ms) (Hahn, E.L. (1950)) and the application of continuous secondary irradiation at the water frequency. The Hahn spin-echo sequence was repeated 128 times for each sample. Spectra were referenced to external sodium-3-(trimethylsilyl)-1-propane-sulphonate (δ = 0ppm).

RESULTS

^{1}H Hahn spin-echo NMR analysis of urine from animals treated with auranofin provided evidence for the induction of nephrotoxic lesions by this novel second-line therapeutic agent (Figure 1). Aminoaciduria was evident by the presence of relatively intense alanine, isoleucine and valine-CH_3 group resonances in spectra of urine obtained from auranofin-treated rats. Moreover, ^{1}H NMR urinalysis also revealed a mild lactic aciduria, as determined by significant rises in the urinary lactate concentrations at time points of 12 and 24 hr. after dosing.

Further modifications in the ^{1}H NMR urine profile included (1) the appearance of ethanol-CH_3 and -CH_2- group resonances, attributable to the gold(I)-blockage of a critical thiol group in the enzyme alcohol dehydrogenase, giving rise to its inhibition; (2) increases in acetate levels; (3) marked decreases in the urinary concentrations of citrate (hypocitraturia) which may be attributable to auranofin-induced modifications in tubular acid-base status and/or effects on the Kreb's cycle; (4) a severe depletion of urinary 2-oxoglutarate; (5) the appearance of resonances attributable to the ketone bodies 3-D-hydroxybutyrate and acetone, the former being of very high intensity. No evidence for glycosuria, nor changes in the urinary levels of trimethylamine N-oxide, dimethylamine and N,N-dimethylglycine was obtained.

^{1}H NMR analysis of plasma obtained from rats both prior and subsequent to auranofin treatment demonstrated drug-induced elevations in the concentrations of alanine, 3-D-hydroxybutyrate and succinate, with decreases in the levels of formate (Figure 2).

The increase in the plasma concentration of 3-D-hydroxybutyrate, together with its corresponding urinary excretion, indicates a high utilisation of fats for energy in auranofin-treated rats. Consistent with this hypothesis, the plasma lipid resonances were diminished in intensity following auranofin treatment. In addition, ethanol was detectable in the plasma samples obtained at 12 and 24 hrs. after dosing.

Since formate can be derived from reactive oxygen radical-mediated oxidative damage to endogenous carbohydrate systems (Grootveld et al (1990a)), the effective suppression of its plasma level in rats by auranofin may be a reflection of the ability of this agent to directly or indirectly control such oxidative damage *in vivo* (Grootveld et al (1990b)).

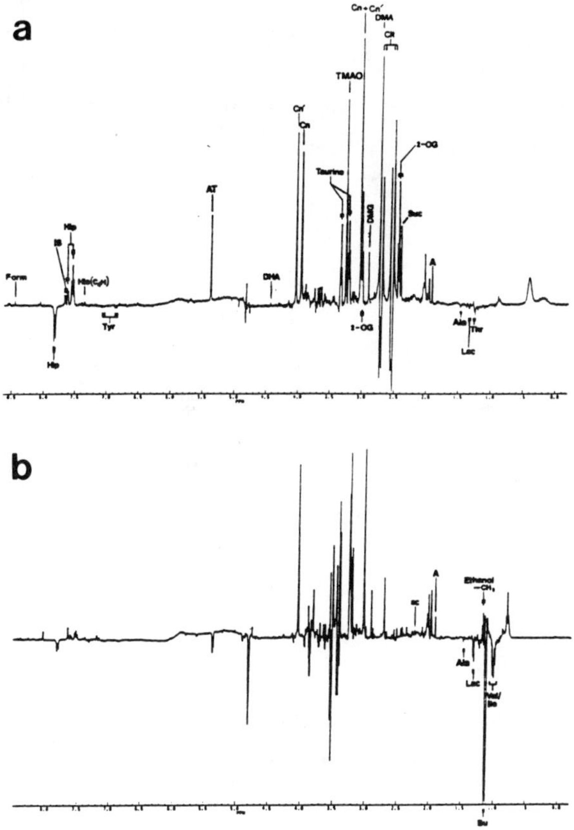

Figure 1 400-MHz ^1H Hahn spin-echo NMR spectra of urine samples obtained from a rat (a) before and (b) 24 hr. after treatment with an intramuscular dose of Auranofin (99 mg/kg). Typical spectra are shown. Abbreviations: A, acetate-CH_3; ac, acetone-CH_3; Ala, alanine-CH_3; AT, allantoin-CH; Bu, 3-D-hydroxybutyrate-CH_3; Cit, citrate-CH_2; Cn, creatinine N-CH_3 and -CH_2- resonances; Cn′, creatine N-CH_3 and -CH_2- group resonances; DHA, dihydroxyacetone-CH_2; DMA, dimethylamine N-CH_3; DMG, N,N-dimethylglycine N-CH_3; Form, formate-H; Hip, hippurate aromatic proton resonances; His(C_4H), histidine C_4-H; Ile, isoleucine-CH_3; IS, indoxyl sulphate aromatic proton resonances; Lac, lactate-CH_3; 2-OG, 2-oxoglutarate -CH_2- group resonances; Suc, succinate-CH_2; TMAO, trimethylamine N-oxide N-CH_3; Thr, threonine-CH_3; Val, valine-CH_3's.

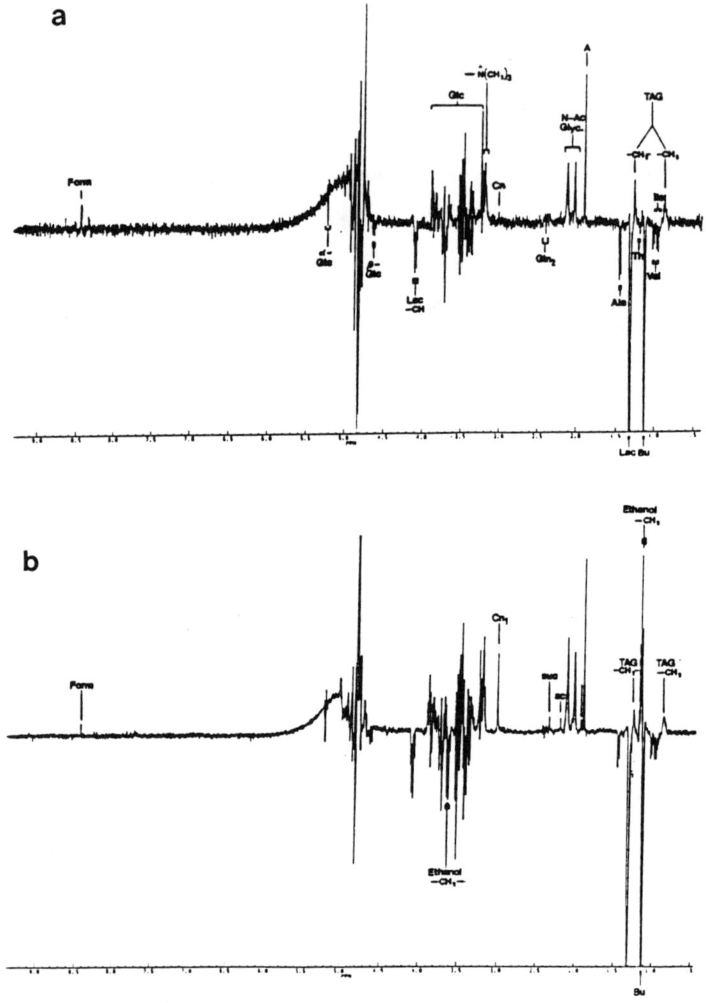

Figure 2 400-MHz ^{1}H Hahn spin-echo NMR spectra of plasma samples obtained from a rat (a) before and (b) 24 hr. after treatment with an intramuscular dose of Auranofin (99 mg/kg). Typical spectra are shown. Abbreviations: as in Fig. 1, with Glc, glucose resonances; α-Glc, glucose α-anomeric proton resonance; β-Glc, glucose β-anomeric proton resonance; Gln_2, $-CH_2$ group of glutamine; Lac-CH, lactate-CH; N-Ac-Glyc., N-acetyl-CH_3 groups of mobile portions of N-acetylated glycoproteins; $-^+N(CH_3)_3$, choline-$^+N(CH_3)_3$ group; TAG-CH_3 and $-CH_2-$, triacylglycerol terminal $-CH_3$ and $-CH_2-$ groups respectively.

DISCUSSION

Parenterally-administered auranofin appears to induce a pattern of proximal tubular kidney damage in rats, consisting of aminoaciduria, lactic aciduria and elevated urinary acetate levels. However, no evidence for glycosuria was obtained in this study. Markiewicz et al (1988) found that auranofin induced a nephropathy in rats which was characterised by acute coagulative necrosis, subacute renal cortical fibrosis, chronic cytomegaly and karyomegaly, and renal cortical neoplasia in the latter stages.

The lactic aciduria, hypocitraturia and detection of ethanol in urine from rats treated with auranofin has previously been observed in animals treated with the nephrotoxin mercury(II) chloride (Nicholson et al (1985)). Interestingly, the aurocyanide anion complex ($[Au^{I}(CN)_2]^-$) has been shown to be a potent inhibitor of liver alcohol dehydrogenase (Gunnarsson and Pettersson (1974)). This inhibition appears to involve the binding of $[Au^{I}(CN)_2]^-$ to the enzyme with the retention of the CN^- ligands on gold(I).

In addition to the auranofin-induced modifications in the concentrations of 3-D-hydroxybutyrate in urine and plasma, and triacylglycerols in plasma, the increased urinary acetate levels may also reflect the effect of auranofin on fatty acid oxidation.

These results demonstrate the application of high-field ^1H NMR spectroscopy for the detection and quantification of abnormal metabolites which are markers of drug-induced renal damage.

Acknowledgements

We are very grateful to the Arthritis and Rheumatism Council for financial support, the University of London Intercollegiate Research Services for the provision of NMR facilities, and to Lin Wells for typing the manuscript.

REFERENCES

Grootveld, M., Henderson, E.B., Farrell, A., Blake, D.R., Parkes, H.G. and Haycock, P. (1990a). Biochem. J. In Press.

Grootveld, M., Blake, D.R., Sahinoglu, T., Claxson, A.W.D., Mapp, P., Stevens, C., Allen, R.E. and Furst, A. (1990b). Free Rad. Res. Commun. In Press.

Gunnarsson, P.-O. and Petterson, G. (1974). Eur. J. Biochem., 43, 474-486.

Hahn, E.L. (1950). Phys. Rev., 80, 580.

Markiewicz, V.R., Saunders, L.Z., Creus, R.J., Payne, B.J. and Hook, J.B. (1988). Fundam. Appl. Toxicol., 11(2), 277-284.

Nicholson, J.K., Timbrell, J.A. and Sadler, P.J. (1985). Mol. Pharmacol. 27, 644-651.

AAS 32
Drugs in Inflammation

INFLUENCE OF AN INTRAVENOUS DOSE OF AUROTHIOMALATE ON THE STATUS OF LOW-MOLECULAR-MASS ENDOGENOUS METABOLITES IN BLOOD PLASMA: A PROTON NUCLEAR MAGNETIC RESONANCE (NMR) STUDY

Martin GROOTVELD*, Andrew W.D. CLAXSON, Declan NAUGHTON, Mike WHELAN, Alexandra FURST and David R. BLAKE

The Inflammation Group, The London Hospital Medical College, London, E1 2AD, U.K.

*Author to whom correspondence should be addressed.

SUMMARY

The effect of aurothiomalate on the status of a wide range of low-molecular-mass endogenous metabolites in blood plasma obtained from animals treated with an intravenous dose of this second-line agent (150 mg/kg) has been assessed by high field proton Hahn spin-echo NMR spectroscopy. As well as modulating the effective concentrations of NMR-detectable biomolecules, aurothiomalate induces a time-dependent decrease in plasma levels of triacylglycerols with a corresponding elevation in the concentration of the ketone body 3-D-hydroxybutyrate, indicating an increased utilisation of fats for energy in rats treated with this 1:1 gold(I)-thiolate complex. These observations may reflect the toxic side-effects that are associated with aurothiomalate treatment.

INTRODUCTION

Oligomeric 1:1 gold(I)-thiolate drugs such as disodium aurothiomalate have been used successfully for many years in the treatment of rheumatoid synovitis, frequently inducing suppression of the disease rather than simply reducing its progress. The usual dosage is equivalent to 30-50 mg of metallic gold per week (administered parenterally), the whole course of treatment usually involving a total of 2 g of gold.

1:1 Gold(I)-thiolate drugs are presumed to have an intracellular site of action since the gold is eventually localised in intracellular organelles (Ghadially et al (1976), Vernon-Roberts et al (1976)). Although neither oligomeric aurothiomalate nor protein cysteinate-bound gold(I) are likely to undergo cellular uptake except by phagocytosis or pinocytosis, it is possible that certain monomeric bis-thiolato complexes (generated by biotransformation of 1:1 gold(I)-thiolates) may be taken up by specific 'target' cells.

We have employed high field proton Hahn spin-echo NMR spectroscopy to elucidate the role of disodium aurothiomalate (Myocrisin) in mediating the status of a wide range of low-molecular-mass endogenous metabolites in blood plasma obtained from animals treated with an intravenous dose of this novel second-line therapeutic agent.

MATERIALS AND METHODS

Animals and treatment A group of male Wistar albino rats (n = 5) were treated with disodium aurothiomalate which was administered intravenously as Myocrisin (100 mg/ml) to give a dose level of 150 mg/kg for each rat. Food and tap water were allowed *ad libitum*. Blood plasma was sampled immediately before and at time points of 15, 90 and 130 min. after dosing.

^{1}H NMR analysis NMR measurements were performed on a Bruker WH 400 spectrometer operating in quadrature detection mode at 400 MHz for ^{1}H. All spectra were recorded at a probe temperature of 25°C. Typically, 0.55 ml of plasma was placed in a 5 mm diameter NMR tube, and 0.07 ml of deuterium oxide (D_20) was added to provide a field-frequency lock. The intense water signal and the broad protein resonances were suppressed by a combination of the Hahn spin-echo sequence (Hahn, E.L. (1950)) and the application of continuous secondary irradiation at the water frequency. The Hahn spin-echo sequence (90°-τ-180°-τ-collect) was repeated 128 times with τ = 60 ms. Chemical shifts were referenced to external sodium 3-(trimethylsilyl)-1-propane sulphonate (TSP).

RESULTS

Proton Hahn spin-echo NMR analysis of plasma samples obtained both prior and subsequent to treatment with disodium aurothiomalate revealed time-dependent decreases in the intensities of the triacylglycerol terminal -CH_3 and -CH_2- group proton resonances with increases in the intensity of the 3-D-hydroxybutyrate-CH_3 group signal, consistent with an increased metabolism of fats for fuel in aurothiomalate-treated rats (Figure I). Moreover, there was also a marked elevation in the glucose:lactate concentration ratio (measured as the ratios of the intensities of the α- or β- anomeric proton resonances of glucose to those of the lactate -CH_3 or -CH signals) which increased with increasing time.

In addition, the previously undetectable AB coupling pattern of citrate resonances became clearly visible at a time point of 130 min. (Figure I), indicating that negatively-charged aurothiomalate displaces this endogenous metabolite from plasma protein binding sites or, alternatively, mediates its release from cellular systems in a time-dependent manner.

Further modifications in the ^{1}H NMR plasma profiles included time-dependent decreases in the intensities of the proton resonances of acetate, alanine,

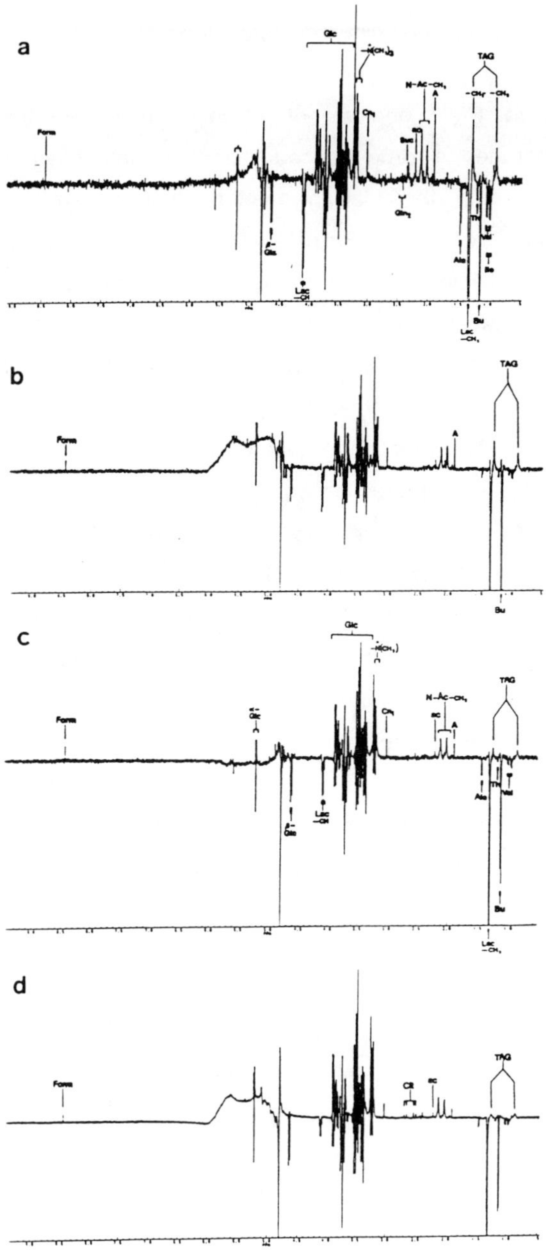

Figure 1 400 MHz ^1H Hahn spin-echo NMR spectra of plasma samples obtained from a rat (a) before and at (b) 15 min., (c) 90 min. and (d) 130 min. after treatment with an intravenous dose of disodium aurothiomalate (150 mg/kg) as 'Myocrisin'. Typical spectra are shown. Abbreviations: A, acetate-CH_3; ac, acetone-CH_3; Ala, alanine-CH_3; Bu, 3-D-hydroxybutyrate-CH_3; Cit, citrate-CH_2; Cn, creatinine-N-CH_3; Form, formate-H; Glc, glucose resonances; α-Glc, glucose α-anomeric proton resonance; β-Glc, glucose β-anomeric proton resonance; Gln_2, -CH_2 group of glutamine; Ile, isoleucine-CH_3; Lac-CH_3 and Lac-GH, lactate -CH_3 and -CH groups; N-Ac-CH_3, N-acetyl-CH_3 groups of mobile portions of N-acetylated glycoproteins; -$^+N(CH_3)_3$, choline-$^+N(CH_3)_3$ group; Suc, succinate-CH_2; TAG-CH_3 and -CH_2-, triacylglycerol terminal -CH_3 and -CH_2- groups respectively; Th, threonine-CH_3; Val, valine-CH_3.

creatinine, formate, glutamine, isoleucine and threonine.

DISCUSSION

High field proton NMR analysis of plasma obtained from rats treated with aurothiomalate demonstrated a drug-induced increased catabolism of fatty acids (i.e., time-dependent decreases in the triacylglycerol resonances and marked increases in the 3-D-hydroxybutyrate-CH_3 group signal). These marked elevations in fatty acid oxidation may arise by interference with oxidative decarboxylation of pyruvate to form acetyl coenzyme A (acetyl CoA) which is catalysed by the pyruvate dehydrogenase complex (Randle, P.J. (1978)). It is possible that this interference occurs by either (a) blockage of the critical thiol (-SH) group in the coenzyme A (CoA) substrate, preventing its conversion to acetyl CoA via the lipoyl acetyltranserase (LAT) enzyme subunit, (b) interaction of gold(I) with the thiol group in the acetyllipoamide form of LAT inhibiting its reaction with the CoA substrate, or (c) blockage of one or both of the essential -SH groups of the dihyrolipoamide form of LAT, preventing its re-oxidation to the lipoamide via the dihydrolipoyl dehydrogenase/FAD system. Gold(I) has a selective high affinity for thiolate sulphur-donor ligands, and in chemical model systems aurothiomalate readily retards the rate of reaction of low-molecular-mass thiols with an aromatic organic disulphide (Grootveld, M. (1985)).

The marked time-dependent increases in the plasma glucose:lactate ratio of aurothiomalate-treated rats indicates a drug-induced gluconeogenesis, and further experiments to assess this are currently in progress.

These results demonstrate the value of proton Hahn spin-echo NMR spectroscopy in assessing the ability of anti-inflammatory drugs to induce changes in the metabolic profile of biological fluids *in vivo*. The aurothiomalate-mediated modifications in rat plasma profile described here are likely to be related to the ability of 1:1 gold(I)-thiolate drugs to induce toxic side-effects (e.g., nephrotoxicity (Vaamonde and Hunt (1970))) in patients treated with these novel therapeutic agents.

Acknowledgements

We are very grateful to the Arthritis and Rheumatism Council for financial support, the University of London Intercollegiate Research Services for the provision of NMR facilities, and to Lin Wells for typing the manuscript.

REFERENCES

Ghadially, F.N., Pruscjal, A.F. and Mitchell, D.M. (1976). Ann. Rheum. Dis., 35, 67.
Grootveld, M. (1985). Ph.D. Thesis, University of London.
Hahn, E.L. (1950). Phys. Rev. 80, 580.
Randle, P.J. (1978). TIBS, Oct., 217-219.
Vaamonde, C.A. and Hunt, F.R. (1970). Arthr. and Rheum. 13(6), 826-834.

INFLUENCE OF DISODIUM AUROTHIOMALATE ON THE ACTIVITIES OF XANTHINE DEHYDROGENASE AND XANTHINE OXIDASE IN ENDOTHELIAL CELLS

Tulin SAHINOGLU , Martin GROOTVELD*, Cliff R. STEVENS , Stephen J. THOMPSON , Andrew W.D. CLAXSON and David R. BLAKE
Inflammation Group, The London Hospital Medical College, London, E1 2AD, UK.
* Author to whom correspondance should be addressed.

SUMMARY

The effect of aurothiomalate in modulating the conversion of xanthine dehydrogenase to its superoxide producing oxidase form in rat and human liver cytosolic preparations has been investigated. Low concentrations (10^{-8}-10^{-5} mol.dm^{-3}) of this second-line agent were found to inhibit the conversion of the dehydrogenase to its corresponding oxidase form. High concentrations (10^{-4} mol.dm^{-3}), however, accelerated this conversion. It is possible that the influence of aurothiomalate on the relative proportions of xanthine dehydrogenase and xanthine oxidase is a reflection of the gold(I) blockage of critical thiol(ate) or sulphido ligands present in this enzymatic system. These effects may form the basis of aurothiomalate's anti-proliferative action on endothelial cells.

INTRODUCTION

The Pathogenesis of ischæmia/reperfusion injury in human tissues has been attributed to the deleterious production of oxygen-derived free radical species (McCord (1987), Halliwell (1987)). Oxygen-derived free radicals, such as the hydroxyl radical ($^{\cdot}OH$) and its precursor, superoxide ($O_2^{\cdot-}$), can contribute to tissue injury, since they have been shown to initiate radical chain reactions that give rise to lipid peroxidation and membrane damage.

A mechanism involving ischæmic/reperfusion injury has previously been suggested to account for the unusual persistence of inflammation in rheumatoid synovium (Woodruff *et al* (1986)). In this hypothesis, the enzyme xanthine oxidase has been postulated to play a pivotal role since it is established that the non-radical producing enzyme xanthine dehydrogenase is converted to the superoxide-producing oxidase form during post-ischæmic reperfusion. The presence of the enzyme in human synovium has been previously reported (Allen *et al* (1987)).

Della Corte and Stirpe (1972) have shown that the conversion of the dehydrogenase ('D') form of the enzyme to the oxidase ('O') form involves the inactivation of one or more functionally important thiol groups. However, the precise chemical nature of these inactivations remain unclear. Consideration of the importance of the modulation of the reactivity of xanthine dehydrogenase thiol groups therefore implicates a potential mechanism of action for the widely used anti-arthritic gold(I)-thiolate drugs. Oligomeric 1:1 gold(I) thiolate complexes (e.g: aurothiomalate [Myocrisin] and aurothiopropanolsulphonate [Allochrysine]) have been used for the treatment of rheumatoid arthritis for many years. However, the structural nature of these compounds and their related chemistry have only recently been investigated (Grootveld *et al* (1984)). Gold(I) is known to have a high affinity for thiolate sulphur-donor ligands and is thus expected to be distributed primarily amongst protein and non-protein thiol groups *in vivo*, and studies of the molecular pharmacology of gold drugs have revealed that this is indeed the case (Rayner *et al* (1989)). Hence, the various postulates that have been put forward to explain the delayed, favourable response obtained following the parenteral administration of these novel therapeutic agents are predominantly those which directly or indirectly involve their ability to block thiol group reactivity.

The effects of these drugs on endothelial cell proliferation is of particular importance in studies of rheumatoid synovitis since angiogenesis is the key phenomenon in the maintainance of pannus growth in these conditions.

In the present paper we have investigated the interaction of disodium aurothiomalate with the xanthine oxidoreductase system. Specifically, we have studied the influence of this therapeutic agent on the relative activities of the 'D' and 'O' forms of the enzyme in rat and human liver cytosolic preparations, since the liver is known to be a rich source of the enzyme.

MATERIALS AND METHODS

Reagents

Xanthine, ß-nicotinamide adenine dinucleotide (NAD^+), the protease inhibitors N-p-tosyl-L-arginine methyl ester (TAME) and phenyl methyl sulphonyl fluoride (PMSF) and bovine serum albumin (BSA) were all purchased from Sigma Chemical Co. Disodium aurothiomalate was generously provided by Rhone Poulenc Ltd. (Dagenham, UK).

Preparation of rat liver homogenates

Male Wistar rats (weight ≈ 250g) were killed by aortal exsanguination under CO_2 anaesthesia followed by cervical dislocation.The liver was removed and immediately placed in 20ml of cold Tris-HCl buffer (0.1. mol.dm^{-3}, pH 8.2), containing 1.00 x 10^{-4} mol.m^{-3} PMSF and 1g dm^{-3} TAME. All procedures were conducted on ice. The liver was then weighed and the appropriate volume of Tris-HCl buffer was added to achieve a 25% preparation (4ml of buffer for 1g of tissue). The liver was scissor minced and homogenised using an electronic homogeniser. The homogenate was then centrifuged at 4°C for 20 min at 2000 rpm. The supernatant from this centrifugation was subjected to further centrifugation for 1 hr at 38,000 rpm. The clear supernatant beneath the fatty upper layer was retained and passed down a pre-packed, Sephadex G-25 column (Pharmacia), eluting with 1% (w/v) BSA in 0.9% (w/v) NaCl with PMSF and TAME as above. This procedure removes low-molecular mass substrates and inhibitors.

Spectrophotometric assay for Xanthine Oxidase

The xanthine oxidase/dehydrogenase activity of the supernatant was then measured spectrophotometrically by following the production of urate from its absorbance at 292 nm, according to the procedure of Waud and Rajagopalan (1976).

RESULTS

The effect of increasing concentrationsof disodium aurothiomalate on the xanthine dehydrogenase activity in both rat and human liver cytosolic preparations are given in Table 1. These data demonstrate that at low concentrations, aurothiomalate inhibits the transformation of the 'D' form of the enzyme to its 'O' form, whereas at high concentrations (ca. 10^{-4} mol.dm^{-3}) the conversion is enhanced. The total enzymatic activity was not affected by aurothiomalate in the concentration range 10^{-8}- 10^{-4} mol.dm^{-3}. Della Corte and Stirpe (1972) found that the organomercurial p-hydroxymercuribenzoate readily accelerated the conversion of the enzyme from the 'D' form to its 'O' form. However, despite the similarities in the chemistry of mercury(II) and gold(I), it should be noted that the reactions of organomercurials with thiolate sulphur-donor ligands have much higher equilibrium constants than those of the reactions of oligomeric 1:1 gold(I) thiolate species with a second equivalent of thiol. Moreover, gold(I)-thiolate complexes exchange thiolate ligands at rapid rates, whilst the corresponding organomercury(II) complexes are kinetically inert.

TABLE I. Influence of increasing concentrations of disodium aurothiomalate (expressed as total gold concentration) on the activity of xanthine dehydrogenase expressed as a percentage of the total enzymatic activity (xanthine dehydrogenase plus xanthine oxidase) in (a) rat and (b) human liver homogenates. All values are the means of two separate determinations. The effect of increasing concentrations of disodium aurothiomalate on the total enzymatic activity of xanthine oxidoreductase (xanthine dehydrogenase plus xanthine oxidase) in rat and human liver homogenates is given in (c). Values are expressed in terms of 10^{-3} units of enzyme/100 mg tissue. All enzymatic activities were inhibitable by 10^{-6} mol.dm^{-3} allopurinol.

[Au(I)]/ mol. dm^{-3}	0	10^{-8}	10^{-7}	10^{-6}	10^{-5}	10^{-4}
(a)	73	68	69	67	69	15
(b)	71	70	71	71	68	15

Total enzyme activity (10^{-3}U/100 mg liver)

(c)	10^{-8}	10^{-7}	10^{-6}	10^{-5}	10^{-4}
Rat					
Control	45	47	49	46	44
Test	45	50	47	46	41
Human					
Control	32	32	34	35	30
Test	35	32	37	34	30

DISCUSSION

Angiogenesis, the process of generation of new blood vessels which requires local endothelial cell (EC) proliferation, is one of the prominent characteristics of synovitis in rheumatoid arthritis. The unusual persistence of inflammation in the synovium of rheumatoid patients is therefore critically dependent on this process.

It appears that the initial stage of the sequence of events that lead to EC proliferation is mediated by a number of cytokines released by infiltrating inflammatory cells (macrophages, PMN's, T- and B-lymphocytes (Matsubara and Ziff (1986)) and it has been speculated that the induction of angiogenesis by these soluble factors is mediated by the resultant increased production of O_2^- from EC. The enzyme xanthine oxidase has been shown to be the major source of O_2^- production in EC. A mediator-induced activation of this enzyme in EC has also been reported (Friedl *et al* (1989)). Although the production of such damaging reactive oxygen species (ROS) has frequently been associated with endothelial cell death, it is somewhat unlikely that such an intrinsic 'suicide' mechanism is operative in these systems. Experimental evidence suggests that the process of O_2^- generation under pathophysiological conditions provides EC with a means of inducing their own proliferation in an attempt to repair the damage initiated by external factors. It appears that the O_2^- generated can 'switch on' a number of silent oncogenes which lead to proliferation of EC (Mantovani and Dejana (1989)). However, if the external insult is continuous and excessive, the intrinsic anti-oxidant enzyme systems are fully saturated giving rise to irreversible damage and cell death.

It has previously been reported that Gold(I)-thiolate drugs, which have been extensively used in the treatment of rheumatoid arthritis, can inhibit EC proliferation in-vitro (Matsubara and Ziff (1987)). We have detected and identified gold deposits in human umbilical vein EC in culture (which had been treated with disodium aurothiomalate) with the use of electron microscopic and electron probe X-ray microanalytical techniques. We have also established that one of the gold(I) thiolate drugs disodium aurothiomalate (Na_2AuStm), at therapeutically-relevant concentrations, inhibits the conversion of the enzyme xanthine dehydrogenase to xanthine oxidase, and thus O_2^- release. On the other hand, higher concentrations have been observed to accelerate xanthine dehydrogenase to oxidase conversion, thereby increasing the amount of O_2^- production. This excessive production of ROS can lead to endothelial cell death, resulting in the recession of the inflammatory process. It is therefore conceivable, that the favourable effects of chrysotherapy can be partly attributed to the modulation of the activity of the enzyme xanthine oxidase in EC and the resultant ROS generating capacity of these cells.

ACKNOWLEDGEMENTS

We are very grateful to the Arthritis and Rheumatism Council for financial support.

REFERENCES

1. Allen RE, Outhwaite JM, Morris CJ and Blake DR. (1978) *Ann Rheum Dis*; **46:** 843-845.
2. Della Corte E and Stirpe F. (1972) *Biochem J;* **126:** 739-745.
3. Friedl HP, Till GO, Ryan US and Ward PA. (1989) *FASEB J*; **3:** 2512-2518.
4. Grootveld M, Razi T, Sadler PJ. (1984) *Clin Rheum;* **351:** 5.
5. Halliwell B. (1987) *FASEB J;* **1:** 364-385.
6. Mantovani A and Dejana E. (1989) *Immunology Today;* **10(11):** 370-375.
7. Matsubara T and Ziff M. (1986) *J Immunol;* **137:** 3295-3298.
8. Matsubara T and Ziff M. (1987) *J Clin Invest;* **79:** 1440-1446.
9. McCord JM. (1987) *Fed Proc;* **46:** 2402-2406.
10. Rayner MH, Grootveld M and Sadler PJ. (1989) *Clin Pharmacol Res;* **9(6):** 377-383.
11. Waud WR and Rajagopalan KV. (1976) *Arch Biochem Biophys;* **172:** 354-364.
12. Woodruff T, Blake DR, Freeman J, Andrews FJ, Salt P and Lunec J. (1986) *Ann Rheum Dis;* **45:** 608-611.

AAS 32
Drugs in Inflammation

APPLICATION OF A NOVEL 1:1 GOLD(I)-CHROMOPHORIC THIOLATE COMPLEX AS A SPECTROPHOTOMETRIC PROBE FOR THE THIOL-EXCHANGE REACTIONS OF ANTI-ARTHRITIC GOLD DRUGS IN BIOLOGICAL FLUIDS

Martin GROOTVELD*, Andrew W.D. CLAXSON, Alexandra FURST, and David R. BLAKE

Inflammation Group, The London Hospital Medical College, London, E1 2AD

*Author to whom correspondence should be addressed

SUMMARY

An oligomeric 1:1 gold(I) complex of the chromophoric thiol 5-mercapto(2-nitrobenzoate) has been synthesized and applied as a spectrophotometric probe for the thiol-exchange reactions of structurally-analagous 1:1 gold(I)-thiolate drugs. For low-molecular-mass thiols, results were consistent with the initial formation of a monomeric mixed-ligand bis-thiolato gold(I) complex followed by further ligand substitution by excess thiol to produce 5-mercapto(2-nitrobenzoate) and a monomeric bis-thiolato gold(I) complex. For human serum albumin, however, the spectrophotometric changes were only consistent with the binding of gold(I) to its single cysteine residue (Cys-34) with the retention of the 5-mercapto(2-nitrobenzoate) ligand on gold(I).

INTRODUCTION

1:1 gold(I)-thiolate complexes have been used successfully for many years in the treatment of rheumatoid synovitis, frequently inducing remission of the disease rather than simply alleviating its progress. However, the structural nature of these complexes has previously been very poorly defined and it is only within the last ten years that attempts to investigate their chemistry have been conducted (Sadler, P.J. (1982), Grootveld et al (1984)). 1:1 Gold(I)-thiolate complexes are often formulated as simple monomers, [Au(SR)], but it is now clear that these species consist of oligomeric rings or chains with gold(I) achieving linear two-coordination via bridging thiolate sulphur-donor ligands, (Grootveld et al (1984), Grootveld, M. 1985)), i.e., $[Au(SR)]_n$ where n is ~ 6. Many commercial preparations contain a slight molar excess of thiolate over gold(I) (Grootveld et al (1984)).

Gold(I) is a soft Lewis acid with a high affinity for thiolate ligands and a low affinity for nitrogen and oxygen-donor ligands. Thus gold(I) distributes itself primarily amongst protein and non-protein thiol groups *in vivo*. For example, in human plasma where the principal source of thiol groups is albumin (Cys-34), gold(I) (parenterally administered as disodium aurothiomalate ('Myocrisin')) is predominantly albumin-bound, but smaller quantities are bound to immunoglobulins and approximately 5% of the total circulating gold is low-molecular-mass or 'free reactive' gold (Danpure, C.J. (1977), Danpure et al (1979), Rayner et al (1989)).

In the present paper we have explored a novel mechanistic approach to the biotransformation and action of oligomeric 1:1 gold(I)-thiolate drugs in biological matrices by the synthesis and application of a structurally-analogous 1:1 gold(I)-chromophoric thiolate complex (1:1 gold(I)-5-mercapto(2-nitrobenzoate),[1]) as a spectrophotometric probe for their biologically-relevant thiolate exchange reactions. The tautomeric thioquinone of the thiolate ligand employed (equation 1) is intensely coloured (E = 1.415 x 10^4 mol^{-1} dm^3 cm^{-1} at 412 nm (pH 7.40) (Riddles et al (1979)) and hence enables a sensitive spectrophotometric assessment of the equilibria, kinetics and mechanism of these reactions in model systems or biological fluids.

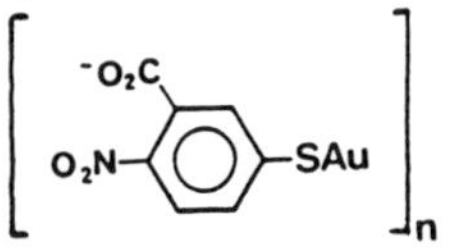

[1]

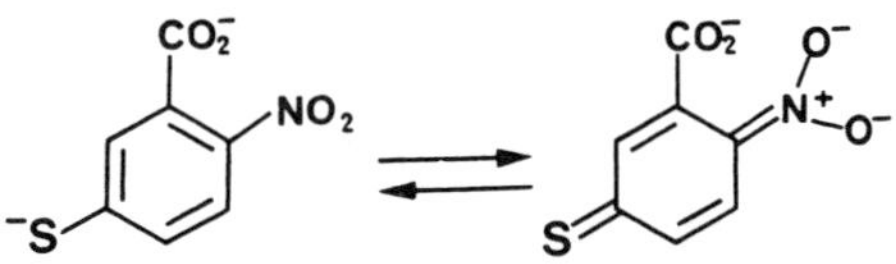

(1)

MATERIALS AND METHODS

Reagents 5,5'-dithiobis(2-nitrobenzoic acid) (DTNB), bis(2-hydroxyethyl) sulphide, thiomalic acid (2-mercaptosuccinic acid), glutathione, cysteine, human serum albumin (HSA) and sodium borohydride ($NaBH_4$) were purchased from Sigma Chemical Co., and sodium tetrachloroaurate(III) dihydrate ($NaAuCl_4.2H_2O$ was a generous gift from Johnson Matthey Research Ltd. (Reading, U.K.). All other chemicals used were of the highest possible grade and obtained from commercially available sources.

Preparation of 1:1 gold(I)-5-mercapto(2-nitrobenzoate)

The 1:1 gold(I)-5-mercapto(2-nitrobenzoate) complex (Au(I)5-MNB) was synthesized by the prior reduction of $[AuCl_4]^-$ to gold(I) with bis(2-hydroxyethyl) sulphide followed by addition of the aromatic thiolate (prepared immediately before by reduction of DTNB with a solution of $NaBH_4$ in ethanol under N_2). Yield, 57%. Elemental analysis: calculated for $AuSC_7H_4O_4N.H_2O$: C, 20.35%; H, 1.46%; N, 3.39%. Found: C, 20.21%; H, 1.46%; N, 3.42%.

Spectrophotometric titrations and kinetic measurements

Spectrophotometric titrations of Au(I)5-MNB with disodium thiomalate, glutathione and cysteine were conducted by the addition of aliquots (5 μl) of thiol stock solutions (in 5.0 x 10^{-2} mol.dm^{-3} phosphate buffer, pH 7.40) to 3.00 ml of a solution of Au(I)5-MNB (containing 4.90 x 10^{-4} mol.dm^{-3} gold) also in 5.0 x 10^{-3} mol.dm^{-3} phosphate buffer (pH 7.40) at a temperature of 37.0°C. Kinetics were monitored spectrophotometrically subsequent to the addition of 20 μl of an Au(I)-5-MNB stock solution (containing 3.00 x 10^{-2} mol.dm^{-3} gold) to 3.00 ml of a 5.00 x 10^{-4} mol.dm^{-3} solution of HSA (in 5.00 x 10^{-2} mol.dm^{-3} phosphate buffer, pH 7.40). Reactions were followed at a temperature of 37.0°C, and all spectra were recorded against a phosphate buffer reagent blank. All spectrophotometric measurements were performed using a Perkin Elmer Lamda-5 spectrophotometer.

RESULTS

Figure 1 shows a spectrophotometric titration of Au(I)5-MNB with increasing concentrations of disodium thiomalate. The decrease in intensity of the broad Au(I)5-MNB sulphur-to-gold(I) charge-transfer absorption band located at 313 nm is accompanied by an increase in absorbance at 412 nm, consistent with the reaction scheme given in equations 2 and 3, where ArS^- represents the thiolate anion (or thioquinone) of 5-mercapto(2-nitrobenzoate). The spectro-photometric changes occurring were complete within the time of mixing.

$$1/n[AuSAr]_n + RSH \rightleftharpoons [RS\text{-}Au\text{-}SAr]^- + H^+ \quad (2)$$

$$[RS\text{-}Au\text{-}SAr]^- + RSH \rightleftharpoons [Au(SR)_2]^- + ArS^- + H^+ \quad (3)$$

Two clear isosbestic points at 240 and 346 nm are produced during the titration. The zero-order and corresponding first-derivative (1D) spectra of the products derived from the reaction of Au(I)5-MNB with excess thiomalate revealed an absorption band centred at 412 nm, confirming the presence of the thioquinone resonance form of 5-MNB following its thiomalate-mediated release from gold(I). Similar spectrophotometric changes were also obtained with the low-molecular-mass endogenous thiols glutathione and cysteine. These reactions were also rapid, being complete within the time of mixing.

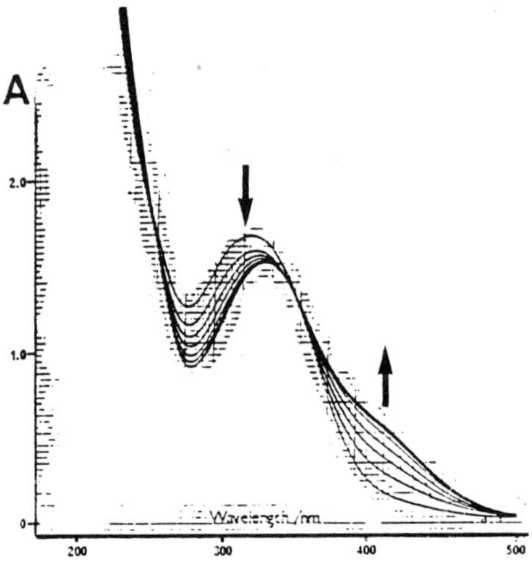

Figure 1

Spectrophotometric titration of Au(I)5-MNB (4.40 x 10^{-4} mol.dm^{-3} gold(I)) with increasing concentrations of disodium thiomalate (0.33-1.98 x 10^{-3}mol.dm^{-3}). T = 37°C.

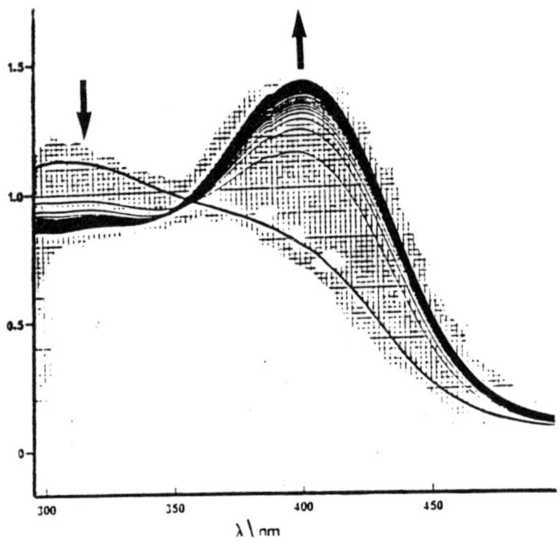

Figure 2

Time-dependent spectrophotometric changes occuring subsequent to the addition of Au(I)5-MNB (1.99 x 10^{-4} mol.dm^{-3} gold(I)) to a 5.00 x 10^{-4} mol.dm^{-3} solution of HSA. Spectra were recorded at 8 min. intervals. T = 37°C.

Figure 2 exhibits the spectrophotometric changes which occur following the addition of Au(I)5-MNB to a 5.00×10^{-4} mol.dm^{-3} solution of HSA. The slow development of an absorption maximum at 402 nm is accompanied by a decrease in intensity of the Au(I)5-MNB band at 313 nm. The absence of an absorption maximum at 412 nm on completion of the reaction (confirmed by 1D spectrophotometry) indicates that 5-MNB is not released from gold(I) during the reaction, and hence for the single thiol group in HSA, the spectrophotometric changes are only consistent with equation 2.

DISCUSSION

These studies demonstrate the value of Au(I)5-MNB as a spectrophotometric probe for the thiolate-exchange reactions of gold(I)-thiolate drugs which occur *in vivo*. In model systems, low-molecular-mass thiols react rapidly with Au(I)5-MNB to form a bis-thiolato gold(I) complex and the thioquinone of 5-MNB, a reaction which proceeds via a mechanism involving a monomeric mixed-ligand bis-thiolato gold(I) complex. However, the single thiol group in HSA reacted with Au(I)5-MNB at a considerably slower rate, reflecting the inaccessibility of its cysteine-34 residue. Application of this novel spectrophotometric probe to biological fluids such as blood plasma or synovial fluid is likely to provide essential clues to our understanding of the kinetics and mechanisms of gold(I)-thiolate biotransformations.

Acknowledgements

We are very grateful to the Arthritis and Rheumatism Council for financial support, and to Lin Wells for typing the manuscript.

REFERENCES

Danpure, C.J. (1977). Proc. Physiol. Soc. 25p.

Danpure, C.J., Fyfe, D.A. and Gumpel, J.M. (1979). Ann. Rheum. Dis. 38, 364.

Grootveld, M.C., Razi, M.T. and Sadler, P.J. (1984). Clin. Rheumatol. 351, 5.

Grootveld, M. (1985). Ph.D. Thesis, University of London.

Rayner, M.H., Grootveld, M. and Sadler, P.J. (1989). Int. J. Clin. Pharm. Res. IX(6), 377-383.

Riddles, P.W., Blakely, R.L. and Zerner, B. (1979). Anal. Biochem. 94, 75.

Sadler, P.J. (1982). J. Rheumatol. 58, 71.

EFFECTS OF AURANOFIN ON ENDOTHELIUM DEPENDENT CONTRACTIONS IN ISOLATED RAT AORTA.

J. Fontaine[1], Z.Y. Fang[2], G. Berkenboom[2] and J.P. Famaey[3].

Laboratory of Pharmacology, Institute of Pharmacy[1], Cardiology Department[2], Erasmus Hospital and Department of Rheumatology[3], Saint-Pierre Hospital, University of Brussels (ULB), Belgium.

SUMMARY : Auranofin (10^{-6} and 10^{-5}M) reduces the acetylcholine induced relaxation in the isolated rat aorta. Contractions induced by phenylephrine and 5-hydroxytryptamine are enhanced by auranofin 10^{-6}M only when endothelium is present. At higher concentration (10^{-5}M), it antagonizes the agonist-induced contractions either in the presence or absence of endothelium.

Auranofin (AUR), an oral gold compound used in the treatment of rheumatoid arthritis has been recently shown to be a potent and selective inhibitor of endothelium-derived relaxing factor (EDRF) in rabbit aorta (Ohlstein and Horohonich, 1989). As a modulatory effect of endothelium on agonist-induced contractions has been demonstrated in various preparations (see Miller et al.,1988),the effects of AUR have been analyzed on the contractile activity of isolated rat aortic strips either with or without endothelium.

MATERIALS AND METHODS.

The experimental set up has been described previously (Fontaine et al., 1984). Concentration-response curves to acetylcholine (ACh) were determined on adjacent rings of the same aorta contracted with phenylephrine (PHE). One ring served as control and was incubated with the solvent (ethanol) for 30 min whereas the other rings were incubated with AUR (10^{-6} or 10^{-5}M) for 30 min.

In order to obtain the same magnitude of contraction in all the preparations (between 1.5 g and 2 g) the dose of PHE varied from 3×10^{-8}M to 10^{-6}M. The IC50 value of ACh measured either in the absence or presence of AUR was defined as the concentration producing 50% decrease of the PHE-induced contraction. In another series of experiments, dose-contraction curves to 5-hydroxytryptamine (5-HT) and PHE were assessed in the continuous presence of propranolol 10^{-6}M (for PHE) or propranolol and phentolamine 10^{-6}M (for 5-HT) in order to avoid interference with α or β adrenoceptor-mediated responses. These curves were reproducible at 60 min intervals. After a first dose-contraction curve (control curve), the preparation was incubated either with the solvent (ethanol)or with AUR 10^{-6} or 10^{-5}M for 30 min and a second curve to the agonist was constructed in their presence. In some preparations, the endothelium was removed by gently rubbing the intimal surface with a cotton pellet. The absence of endothelium was confirmed by the lack of response to ACh (10^{-5}M). The EC50 values of PHE or 5-HT were defined as the concentrations inducing 50% of the maximal response measured in the control curve. Auranofin was a generous gift from Smith Kline Beecham (Rixensart, Belgium).

RESULTS

Effect on ACh-induced relaxations.

AUR 10^{-6}M produced a rightward shift of the concentration response curve to ACh of about 16 : the IC50 increased from $5.0 \times 10^{-8} \pm 0.5$ g to $8.0 \times 10^{-7} \pm 0.6$ g ($n = 6$, $P < 0.001$) and the maximal response was only 61% $\pm$ 3 ($P < 0.001$) of the PHE contraction (versus 87% $\pm$ 4 for the control). In the presence of AUR 10^{-5}M, the IC50 could not be determined, the maximal response to ACh reaching only 42 $\pm$ 6% ($P < 0.001$) of the PHE contraction (fig.1).

Effect on PHE-and 5-HT-induced contractions.

These results are illustrated in fig.2 and Table I. In preparations with endothelium (fig. 2 A-C) AUR 10^{-6}M induced a significant leftward shift of the concentration-response curves to PHE and 5-HT with a decrease in the EC50 of both agonists and a significant increase in the maximal response induced by PHE. In the presence of AUR 10^{-5}M the responses to PHE were significantly decreased at all the concentrations tested while those to 5-HT were increased at the lower concentrations of the agonist and decreased at the higher concentrations. In preparations without endothelium (Fig. 2 B-D) AUR had dose-dependent inhibitory effects on PHE and 5-HT induced contractions.

TABLE I

WITH ENDOTHELIUM		EC50 (M)	shift x	max.response (g)	%
PHE	control	$1.5 \times 10^{-7} \pm 0.5$ (11)	-	2.04 ± 0.19	100
	AUR 10^{-6}	$2.7 \times 10^{-8} \pm 0.7$ (6)*	5.5 (L)	2.70 ± 0.20*	132.2
	AUR 10^{-5}	$7.3 \times 10^{-6} \pm 0.4$ (5)***	48.6 (R)	1.12 ± 0.12**	54.9
5-HT	control	$5.5 \times 10^{-6} \pm 0.7$ (10)	-	2.65 ± 0.19	100
	AUR 10^{-6}	$2.7 \times 10^{-6} \pm 0.5$** (5)	2.0 (L)	3.13 ± 0.32 NS	118.0
	AUR 10^{-5}	$2.0 \times 10^{-6} \pm 0.2$*** (5)	2.7 (L)	2.10 ± 0.13*	79.5
WITHOUT ENDOTHELIUM					
PHE	control	$1.4 \times 10^{-8} \pm 0.5$ (11)	-	2.40 ± 0.19	100
	AUR 10^{-6}	$5.4 \times 10^{-8} \pm 0.9$** (6)	3.8 (R)	2.22 ± 0.18 NS	92.2
	AUR 10^{-5}	- (5)		0.99 ± 0.23**	41.2
5-HT	control	$2.7 \times 10^{-6} \pm 0.6$ (10)	-	2.78 ± 0.16	100
	AUR 10^{-6}	$2.8 \times 10^{-6} \pm 0.5$ NS (5)	1.0	2.25 ± 0.15*	81.0
	AUR 10^{-5}	$7.0 \times 10^{-6} \pm 0.8$** (5)	2.6 (R)	1.82 ± 0.11***	65.4

Results are expressed as means ± S.E., number of experiments in ( )
Student's t test for paired data versus control *** $P < 0.001$ ** $P < 0.01$ * $P < 0.05$
NS : Non significant
x : ratios of EC50 and shifts to the left (L) or right (R)

DISCUSSION

AUR (10^{-6} and 10^{-5}M) dose-dependently inhibits endothelium dependent relaxations induced by ACh in the rat aorta. This confirms the data obtained by Ohlstein and Horohonich (1989) in the rabbit aorta. Moreover, at 10^{-6}M, AUR is able to slightly but significantly potentiate the PHE- and 5-HT-induced contractions.

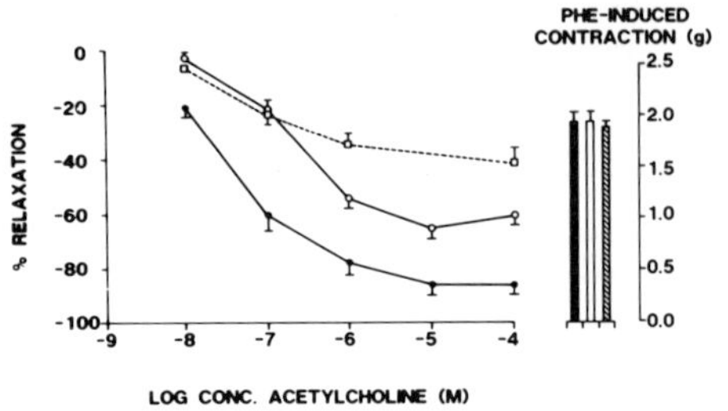

Fig.1 - Concentration-response curves to ACh in the absence (●) and presence of AUR 10^{-6}M (–o–) and 10^{-5}M (--□--). Histograms illustrate the contractions to PHE 10^{-7}M (black columns), 3 x 10^{-8}M + AUR 10^{-6}M (open columns) and 10^{-6}M + AUR 10^{-5}M (hatched columns). Mean values (± SE) refer to 6 individual experiments.

This is in accordance with an impairment of the endothelial function as removal of the endothelium has been shown to potentiate the contractile activity of rat aorta to various agonists (see Miller et al. 1988). These results support the view that AUR is a potent inhibitor of EDRF. As it does not modify the vascular relaxations of rabbit aorta induced by nitric oxide (Ohlstein and Horohonich, 1989) which has a remarkable similarity to action with EDRF (Ignarro, 1989),its effects cannot be explained through inhibition of EDRF effect. Membrane peroxidation in the endothelium with generation of superoxide anion leading to EDRF degradation should be a better explanation of AUR effects (see Snyder et al. 1989). As EDRF was recently suggested to be a nitrosothiol (Myers et al. 1990), an alternative hypothesis should be that AUR reacts with thiol groups (see Snyder et al., 1987) leading to inactivation of EDRF. The effects of AUR in the rat aorta can however not be explained only in terms of EDRF inactivation. Indeed, at concentrations inhibiting greatly the ACh-induced relaxations, AUR (10^{-5}M) exerted inhibitory effects on PHE- and to a lesser extent on 5HT-induced contractions. These inhibitory effects already appear in the presence of AUR 10^{-6}M when the endothelium was removed. In our experimental conditions, the PHE-and 5-HT-induced contractions can be attributed to activation of postjunctional $5HT_2$ receptors and α_1 adrenoceptors resulting in both the entry of extracellular Ca^{2+} and its release from intracellular stores via inositol phospholipid hydrolysis. An interference with the release of intracellular Ca^{2+} at one of the steps following receptors activation should probably be considered to explain the inhibitory effects of AUR on the vascular

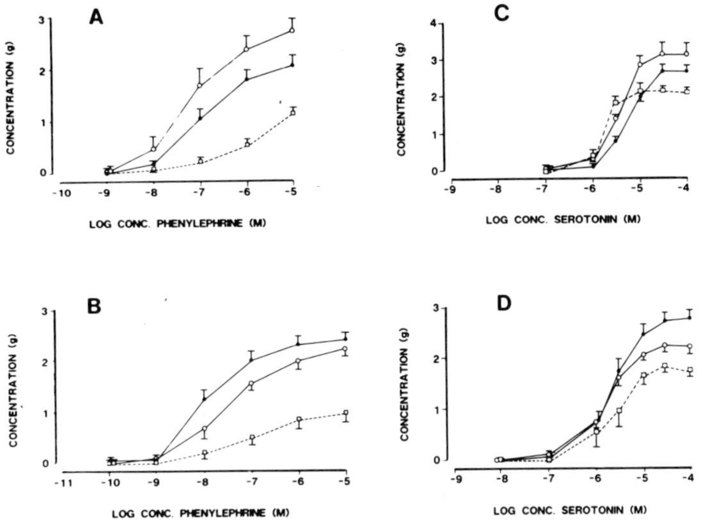

Fig.2 - Effects of AUR 10^{-6}M (—o—) and 10^{-5}M (--□--) on the contractions induced by PHE (●) and 5-HT (●) in aortae with (A and C) and without (B and D) endothelium. Mean values (± SE) refer to 5-6 individual experiments.

contractility. This could occur through activation of adenylate cyclase activity which has been shown in platelets (Winther et al. 1988). This hypothesis should however be further investigated.

REFERENCES

Fontaine, J., Herchuelz, A. and Famaey, J.P. (1984). A pharmacological analysis of the responses of isolated aorta from rats with adjuvant arthritis. Agents and Actions, 14, 684-687.

Ignarro, L.J. (1989). Endothelium derived nitric oxide : actions and properties. FASEB J., 3, 31-36.

Miller, R.C., Schini, V. and Schaeffter, P. (1988). Modulation by the endothelium of agonist-induced contractions of vascular smooth muscle. In : Relaxing and Contracting factors (P.M. Vanhoutte, Ed.), Humana, Clifton, pp. 241-265.

Myers, P.R., Minor Jr. R.L., Guerra Jr. R., Bates, J. and Harrison, D.G. (1990). Vasorelaxant properties of the endothelium-derived relaxing factor more closely resemble S-nitrosocysteine than nitric oxide. Nature, 345, 161-163.

Ohlstein, E.H. and Horohonich, S. (1989). Selective inhibition of endothelium-dependent relaxation by gold-containing compounds. Pharmacology, 38, 93-100.

Snyder, R.M., Mirabelli, C.K. and Crooke, S.T. (1987).The Cellular Pharmacology of Auranofin. Semin. Arthritis. Rheum.,17, 71-80.

Winther, K., Oxholm, P. and Sengelow, H. (1988). Effect of Auranofin on human platelet aggregation, release of serotonin, and cyclic-AMP formation. Inflammation, 12, 107-112.

New Approaches to Pain Relief

AAS 32
Drugs in Inflammation

ELECTROPHYSIOLOGICAL MECHANISMS IN INFLAMMATORY PAIN

H.O. Handwerker
Department of Physiology and Biokybernetics,
University of Erlangen/Nürnberg, Universitätsstraße 17, D-8520
Erlangen
F.R.G.

SUMMARY

Inflammatory pain is mediated from the periphery by a specialized subgroup of nerve fibers, the nociceptors. The nociceptive nerve endings undergo sensitization and excitation when stimulated with inflammatory agents. It will be shown that a multitude of substances cooperates in this process. Since nociceptive nerve endings are too small to be approached directly with the methods of intracellular electrophysiology, one has to extrapolate to the membrane channels and intracellular processes mediating nociceptor sensitization from studies on the pericarya of sensory ganglion cells.
Sustained inflammation induces profound plastic changes in peripheral and central neurones leading to an altered excitability.

INTRODUCTION

Inflammatory pain is mediated by peripheral nerve fibers and by intricately connected central neurons. The code of this information consists of action potentials spreading via axons, and of local postsynaptic potentials which do not only initiate axon potentials in target neurones, but also modulate the neuronal information in various ways.
This neuronal system is in itself incredibly complicated and far from fully understood. However, a proper discussion of the neurophysiology of inflammatory pain is further complicated, since quite different neuronal events may be prominent in different types of acute and chronic inflammation.
Since the author has recently dealt with this subject in detai-

led reviews (Handwerker et al.,1990; Handwerker & Reeh, 1990; Handwerker,1990), only a short survey will be provided in this paper.

Nociceptors in acute inflammation

The peripheral primary afferent nerve fibers mediating the pain induced by a trauma have been called nociceptors. They consist of unmyelinated (C-) and thin myelinated (A-delta) slowly conducting nerve fibers lacking the end organs typical of the mechanoreceptors. Many of these nociceptive nerve fibers synthetize neuropeptides such as substance P and release them from their peripheral and central nerve endings upon stimulation. The release of vasoactive neuropeptides leads to vasodilatation and plasmaextravasation and has been described as "neurogenic inflammation".

Inflammation of the skin and most other tissues is characterized by (a) ongoing pain, and (b) hyperalgesia. In recent years many studies were devoted to the question which changes in nociceptor responsiveness mediate these phenomena. Most often cutaneous inflammation was induced by heating, but also by chemical agents (for a review see Handwerker and Reeh, 1990; Campbell et al., 1989). It has been found that many nociceptive nerve elements become "spontanously" active in the course of the development of an inflammation and this may be a source of ongoing pain. When nociceptors in inflamed tissue are stimulated by heat, their thresholds are lowered and their discharge rates at suprathreshold temperatures are more rigorous. This sensitization may be the neuronal basis of the hyperalgesia to heat stimuli. However, hitherto in cutaneous nociceptors no clear correlate has been found for the mechanical hyperalgesia which is also prominent in inflamed skin.

There is some controversy, whether the sensitization of unmyelinated (C-) or thin myelinated (A-delta) "polymodal" nociceptors is prominent in inflammatory pain. Several studies came to the conclusion that in the primate hairy skin C fibers but not

A delta fibers account for the hyperalgesia after a heat trauma. This notion is supported by the lack of change in the time course of hyperalgesia and its unchanged magnitude during an A-fiber block in a human skin nerve. However, the situation may be different in the glabrous skin of man and other primates where no reliable sensitization of polymodal C units has been found. Hence, in this type of tissue the sensitization of myelinated nociceptors may be responsible for the hyperalgesia (Meyer & Campbell, 1981).

Nociceptors in deep tissues have also been studied, e.g. in the muscle, in knee joints, the bowels and the urinary bladder. The thin afferent nerve fibers in these tissues were also found getting spontaneously active and sensitized in inflammation.

Chemical irritant substances induce changes in nociceptor responsiveness rather similar to those induced by a heat trauma. Some of these substances, e.g. mustard oil and capsaicin, induce predominantly the "neurogenic" type of inflammation, whereas others may lead to inflammatory processes which are rather independent of the nerve supply of the tissue. However, the changes observed in nociceptors seem to be rather similar after application of both types of irritants. usually spontaneous activity and sensitization to heat stimuli is prominent. Often the spontaneous activity is temporarily abolished by moderate cooling.

Mediators of nociceptor sensitization

The nociceptor sensitization is very likely mediated by the various substances released in the course of an inflammation. The highly complex local reactions to tissue injuries often start with an activation of the endothelial cells of the small blood vessels resulting in a perivascular edema. Potent agents are released which affect local immunocompetent cells, e.g. the mast cells, increase the vascular permeability, and excite afferent nociceptive nerve endings from which in turn neuropeptides are released. This acute phase of the inflammatory reaction is followed by the immigration of PMN leukocytes, lymphocytes and monocytes, into the injured tissue. T-lymphocytes and macrophages release another typ of inflammatory agents, the cytokines, which are able to transform other local cells such as fibroblasts into an inflammatory state.

Up to now mainly the effects of the "classical" mediators released in early stages of acute inflammations have been studied with respect to their effect on nociceptor functions. The effects of later stages, and in particular of the cytokines on the nociceptors are largely unknown.

Recently potent in vitro techniques have been developed for the study of the impact of individual agents on afferent nerve endings in mammals (Reeh, 1986; Kumazawa et al., 1987). With these techniques it was found that agents such as bradykinin, histamine and serotonin indeed excite and sensitize nociceptive nerve endings at micromolar concentrations. Furthermore, it has been proven that nociceptive nerve endings are rather sensitive to H^+ concentrations at a pH below 6.9 which has a parallel to the acid pH of inflamed tissue.

In general, these studies on inflammatory agents have not revealed a single chemical principle of nociceptor sensitization. Instead, many endogenous substances seem to condition each other to this effect.

Putative membrane mechanisms and second messengers

Only extracellular recordings can be obtained from A-delta and C-fibers. Furthermore, usually the action potentials are not recorded at the nerve endings themselves, but proximally from axons in nerve stems. Therefore, the exact nature of the transduction mechanisms relating noxious stimuli and membrane processes has not been directly studied. For the analysis of ionic currents other models, e.g. cell bodies in isolated sensory ganglia or small capsaicin-sensitive ganglion cells in culture, have been substituted.

Fig.1 summarizes some of the present ideas on membrane proecesses in nociceptors.

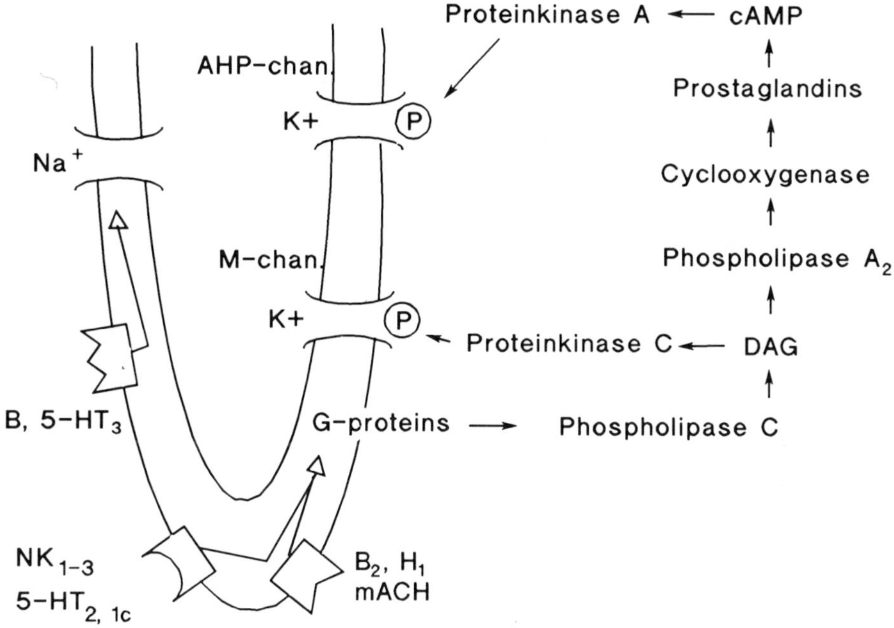

Fig. 1
Putative second messenger mechanisms in nociceptor activation. For details see text.

Several membrane receptors, e.g. the B_2 bradykinin receptor, the muscarinic acetylcholine receptor, the H_1 histamine receptor, the 5-HT_2 receptor and the neurokinin receptors are assumed to induce depolarization by a common second messenger system: proteinkinase C, activated via G proteins, phospholipase C and DAG, phosphorylates and by that closes a K^+ channel, the M-channel (Brown, 1988; Role & Schwarz, 1989). On the other hand, the released DAG is assumed to activate phospholipase A_2 leading, via cyclooxygenase, to the release of prostaglandins E which in turn activate proteinkinase A via cAMP increase. Proteinkinase A has been shown to phosphorylate another K^+ chan-

nel, the Ca^{++} dependent AHP channel (Tsien et al.,1988). According to this hypothesis depolarisation and excitation is mainly due to an inactivation of two K^+ channels.
These second messenger pathways are a rather common feature of many cell types but their role in nociceptors is not yet established, though there is some experimental evidence for a contribution of proteinkinase C (Dray & Perkins, 1988; Dray et al., 1988).
Other mechanisms have also been assumed, e.g. activation of a receptor gated Na^+, or unspecific cation-channel by bradykinin and by $5\text{-}HT_3$ receptors (Rang, 1990).

Repetitive application of inflammatory agents to nociceptive nerve endings usually leads to tachyphylaxis. Fig. 2 shows its hypothetical mechanism.

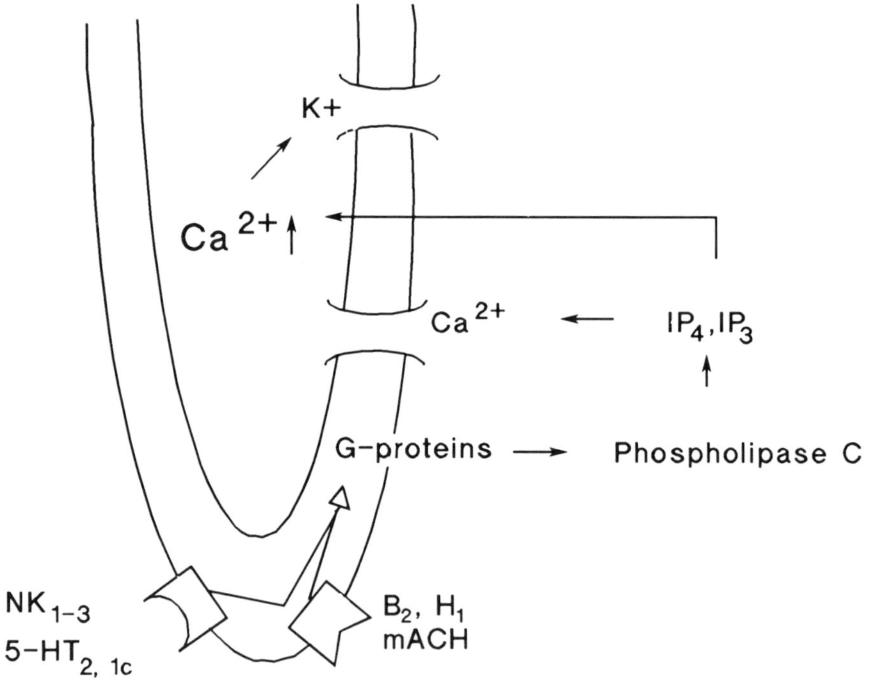

Fig.2
Hypothetical mechanisms of tachyphylaxis. For details see text.

The phospholipase C activates the IP_3 and IP_4 system leading to an increase in intracellular Ca^{++} and hence possibly to an activation of Ca^{++}- dependent K^+ channels (Nahorski, 1988). If this mechanism plays a role in nocicepters, it would counteract excitation and hence provide a hypothetical explanation of the tachyphylaxis. Indeed, it has been found that a lowering of the extracellular Ca^{++} level counteracted BK tachyphylaxis (Lang et al., 1990). However, a unifying hypothesis of the tachyphylaxis does not explain the lack of cross-tachyphylaxis between 5-HT and BK (Beck et al., 1974).

Recruitment of unresponsive nociceptors and plastic changes in primary afferents and in central neurones

Recent evidence suggests that in various tissues, i.e. in the joints, in the urinary bladder, in the colon and in the skin there are many small fiber afferents which under physiological conditions are not responsive even to noxious stimulation, but become activated in inflammation. The conditions of the recruitment of "unresponsive" or "sleeping" nociceptors are still unknown. However, the discovery of this group of afferent nerve fibers has led to the assumption that the population of peripheral nerve units mediating inflammatory pain is quite different from that mediating acute stimulus induced pain.
Evidence is accumulating that inflammatory processes potentiate the plastic alteration of the structure and biochemistry of nociceptors and of central neurones. An example of peripheral plasticity is the increase of the synthesis and of the axonal transport of neuropeptides in small primary afferents in chronic inflammation. Likewise, in inflammation opiate receptors are synthetized in the cell bodies of small afferent nerve fibers at an increased rate and transported to the nerve endings. Examples of central nervous plasticity are the changed responsiveness and enlarged receptive fields of many neurones in the dorsal horn of the spinal cord after exposure to tonic nociceptive input (Woolfe, 1990). These alterations seem to have a structural basis. It has been shown that e.g. the c-fos oncogene is expressed in lamina I and V dorsal horn neurones after prolonged noxious input related to inflammatory states (Menetrey et al., 1989). C-fos protein may induce the synthesis of proenkephaline, prodynorphine and of nerve growth factor in some neurones.

It may be concluded from these recent findings that inflammation induces profound changes in the peripheral and central nervous system reaching beyond the changes in electrical excitability of primary nociceptive afferents observed by means of classical electrophysiology.

REFERENCES

Beck, PW, Handwerker, HO (1974) Bradykinin and serotonin effects on various types of cutaneous nerve fibres. Pflügers Arch. 347:209-222

Brown D, (1988) M-currents: an update. Trends Neurosci., 11: 294-299.

Campbell JN, Raja AN, Cohen RH, Manning DC, Khan AA, Meyer RA (2nd Ed.; 1989) Peripheral neural mechanisms of nociception. In: Textbook of Pain (Wall P D and Melzack R, eds) pp 22-45

Dray A, Bettaney J, Forster P, Perkins MN, (1988) Bradykinin-induced stimulation of afferent fibers is mediated through protein kinase C. Neuroscience Letters, 91:301-308.

Dray A, Perkins MN, (1988) Bradykinin activates peripheral capsaicin-sensitive fibers via a second messenger system. Agents & Actions, 25:214-216.

Handwerker HO (1990) What peripheral mechanisms contribute to nociceptive transmission and hyperalgesia? In: "Towards a new pharmacotherapy of pain". Dahlem Konferenzen.(Basbaum AI; Besson J-M ed.) John Wiley & Sons. Chichester (in press).

Handwerker HO, Reeh PW, Steen KH (1990) Effects of 5HT on nociceptors.1-15.In:Serotonin and Pain.(J.M.Besson ed.) Excerpta Medica. Amsterdam, New York, Oxford

Handwerker HO, Reeh PW (1990) Pain and Inflammation. Adelaide,In:in "Proceedings of the VIth World Congress on Pain" (Pain Research and Clinical Management, Vol.5).(Bond M et al. eds.) Elsevier. North Holland (in press).

Kumazawa T, Mizumura K,Sato J, (1987) Response properties of polymodal receptors studied using in vitro testis superior spermatic nerve preparations of dogs. J. Neurophysiology, 57:702-711.

Lang E, Novak A, Reeh PW, Handwerker HO, (1990) Chemosensitivity of fine afferents from rat skin in vitro. J.Neurophysiol., 63:887-901.

Menetrey, D, Gannon, A, Levine, JD.,Basbaum, AI (1989) Expression of C-Fos Protein in Interneurons and Projection Neurons of the Rat Spinal Cord in Response to Noxious Somatic, Articular, and Visceral Stimulation. J. Comp. Neurol. 285:177-195.

Meyer, RA, Campbell, JN, (1981) Peripheral neural coding of pain sensation. Johns Hopkins APL Technical Digest, 2:164-171.

Nahorski, SR (1988) Inositol polyphosphates and neuronal calium homeostasis. Trends NeuroSci. 11:444-448.

Rang HP (1990) The nociceptive afferent neurone as a target for new types of analgesic drug. Pain, Suppl. 5:S249.

Reeh, PW. (1986) Sensory receptors in mammalian skin in an in vitro preparation. Neurosci. Lett. 66:141-146.

Role L, Schwarz JH (1989) Cross-talk between signal transduction pathways. Trends Neurosci., 12, Centrefold.

Tsien RW,Lipscombe D, Madison DV, Bley KR, Fox FP (1988) Multiple types of neuronal calcium channels and their selective modulation. Trends Neurosci., 11:431-438.

Woolfe CJ (1990) Central mechanisms of acute pain. Pain, Suppl. 5:S218.

AAS 32
Drugs in Inflammation

MOLECULAR BASE OF ACETYLCHOLINE AND MORPHINE ANALGESIA

S.H. Ferreira, I.D.G. Duarte and B.B. Lorenzetti

Department of Pharmacology, Faculty of Medicine of Ribeirão Preto, 14.100- Ribeirão Preto-SP, Brasil.

SUMMARY: We have previously described the peripheral analgesic effect of dibutyryl cyclic GMP, acetylcholine (ACh) and morphine (Mph) injected into the rat paws. Since ACh induces nitric oxide (NO) release from endothelial cells which is though to stimulate guanylate cyclase (GC) we investigated if NO-cyclic GMP pathway was involved in the analgesia by those agents. Using a modification of the Randall-Selitto rat paw test, it was found that sodium nitroprusside, which releases NO non-enzymatically, blocked rat paw PGE_2 induced hyperalgesia. The peripheral analgesic effect of sodium nitroprusside, ACh and morphine was enhanced by intraplantar injection of an inhibitor of cyclic GMP phosphodiesterase (MY5445) and blocked by a GC inhibitor, methylene blue (MB). Peripheral analgesia induced by ACh and morphine, but not by sodium nitroprusside, was blocked by N^G-monomethyl-L-arginine (L-NMMA) an inhibitor of the formation of NO from L-arginine. Central effect of morphine as tested by the rat paw and by the tail flick tests was inhibited by intraventricular injection of methylene blue. In addition, the central morphine analgesia was potentiated by My5445. In contrast, with the periphery, the central effect of morphine was not blocked by L-NMMA. Our results demonstrate that NO causes peripheral analgesia via stimulation of GC and supports the suggestion that at this site morphine and acetylcholine analgesia is subsequent to NO release. In the mechanism of the central analgesic effect of morphine, the cGMP system is activated but via NO release, probably by a direct stimulation of the receptors. This is the first demonstration that links peripheral and central analgesic effect of morphine to the stimulation of GC system.

Morphine (Mph) and acetylcholine (ACh) are known to produce central and peripheral analgesia. Notwithstanding the vast number of studies little is known about the biochemical chain of events linking the receptor binding and the analgesic effect. Negative modulation of adenylatecyclase activity, changes in Ca^{2+} and neuronal membrane composition have been evoked in attempts to establish a possible causal relationship between opiate stimulation and the analgesic central effect (for review, see Ronai and Székely, 1982). In the periphery, Ferreira and Nakamura (1979) described analgesic effect of cholinergic agents, known stimulators of guanylate cyclase (GC) and because dibutyryl cyclic GMP also caused analgesia, we suggested that cholinergic agents might cause analgesia via an increase in cyclic GMP at nociceptor level.

Nitric Oxide (NO), an endothelium-derived relaxing factor (Moncada et al., 1988) is formed by vascular endothelial cells from the terminal guanido nitrogen atoms of the amino acid L-arginine (Palmer et al., 1988a). This biosynthetic process, as well as Ach-induced vasodilatation are inhibited by the L-arginine analogue, N^G-monomethyl-L-arginine, L-NMMA (Palmer et al., 1988b; Rees et al., 1989a). The vasodilator effect of acetylcholine is presently explained by the release of NO and stimulation of the soluble GC (Moncada et al., 1988).

The objective of the present study was to test the hypothesis that GC activation in the periphery by Ach or Mph cause antinociception. For this purpose we have tested, in the rat paw, substances which indirectly stimulate GC (ACh and sodium nitroprusside, SNP). The increase of celular cyclic GMP induced by Ach and Mph was confirmed using MB and MY 5445, inhibitors of GC and cyclic GMP phosphodiesterase, respectively. The participation of NO in Mph- and ACh-induced peripheral analgesia was confirmed using the inhibitor of the NO biosyntetic pathway, L-NMMA.
In the present investigation male Wistar rats (130-180 g) were used to measure the intensity hyperalgesia by mean of a modification of the Randall-Selitto rat paw pressure test (Ferreira et al., 1978) and central analgesia by mean of the tail-flick test (Azani et al., 1982) .

RESULTS AND DISCUSSION: ACh (50 to 200 μg/paw) and SNP (50 to 500 μg/paw) caused a dose-dependent analgesia. The control intensity of hyperalgesia changed from 19 sec in paws sensitized with PGE_2 to 9-10 s. The intraplantar injection of the highest dose of ACh or SNP did not affect the PG-induced hyperalgesia in the contralateral paws, thus, indicating that the effect is restricted to the treated paws. In order to test the involvement of the cGMP system, the rat paws were pretreated with MB (500 μg/paw) or MY5445 (50 μg/paw) 1 h before the intraplantar injections of Ach, SNP or Mph. MB significantly inhibited and MY5445 potentiated the peripheral analgesic effects of ACh, SNP and Mph. Neither MB nor MY5445 had any effect upon PG induced hyperalgesia. In order to test if the analgesic effects of ACh, SNP or Mph were direct or mediated via NO release the paws were pretreated with L-NMMA, an inhibitor of the biosynthetic pathway for NO production (Palmer et al., 1988b). Intraplantar injections of L-NMMA (50 μg/paw) abolished the peripheral analgesic effect of ACh and Mph but did not affect that of SNP. These results suggest that both Ach and Mph are producing peripheral analgesia by activating arginine-NO pathway. D-NMMA in identical conditions had no inhibitory effects. Considering several similarities between the peripheral and central effect of ACh and Mph analgesia (Ferreira et al., 1983), we investigated if the same biochemical pathways were involved in morphine central effect. This hypothesis was tested by injecting MB into the cerebral ventricles of rats which received a dose of Mph (8 mg/kg/ip). We have previously shown that this dose of morphine to mainly have a central effect, since quaternary nalorphine was able to antagonize only 8% of its effect (Lorenzetti & Ferreira, 1987). Figure 1 shows that in the modified Randall Selitto test as well the tail flick test, MB pretreatment gave identical results upon morphine induced analgesia. Thus, indicating that the central analgesic effect of Mph is related to an activation of cGMP system. This suggestion was supported using an inhibitor of cyclic GMP phosphodiesterase. MY5445 (50 μg) strongly potentiated the central effects of systemically given Mph (1,2,4 mg/kg/ip). The next question was if the central effect of morphine was mediated by NO release. A very small antagonism of L-NMMA against systemically administered Mph (8 mg/kg, rat paw pressure test) was detected. This antagonism was probably peripheral, since intraventricular injections of L-NMMA, even in larger doses than that which abolished the intraplantar

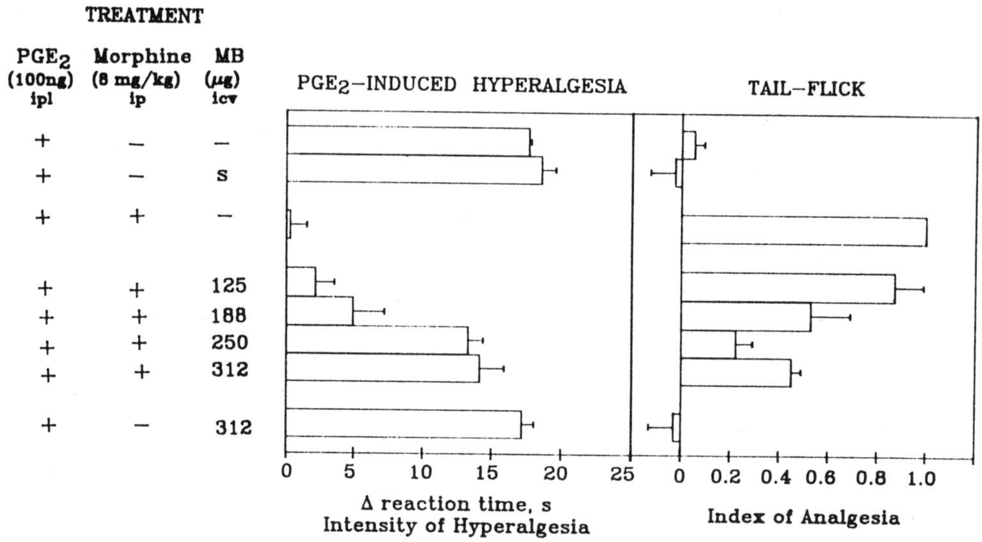

Fig. 1- Blockade by intracerebroventricular (ICV) injection of methylene blue (MB) of morphine central analgesia upon PGE2 induced rat paw hyperalgesia and tail flick tests.
LEFT PANEL: The intensity of rat paw hyperalgesia was measured (delta reaction time, s) 3h after PGE2 (100 ng) intraplantar administration. Morphine treatment (8mg/kg,ip) was made 2 hours after PGE2 challenge. Methylene blue (MB) was injected, icv, 1 hour before morphine. RIGHT PANEL: The tail flick latency measurements were made in the same rat just after the PG hyperalgesia measurements. S= ICV injection of saline . Each bar represents the mean ± S.E.M. of 5 animals.

analgesic effect of Mph, showed no analgesia (both methods). These results, in contrast with those of intraplantar injections, indicate that L-NMMA does not affect Mph central analgesia.

In conclusion, we have provided evidences for NO-cyclic GMP pathway in peripheral analgesia of ACh and Mph. The absence of effect of L-NMMA upon morphine central analgesia may be interpreted considering that L-NMMA given systemically or into the cerebral ventricles is unable to reach the sites of analgesic action of morphine or alternatively, morphine central activation of the guanylate system is independent of NO release. In this context, is interesting to note that there are two basic mechanisms of activation of the GC system. One is by activation of soluble GC carried out by nitrovasodilators and free radicals (nitric oxide) and the other, is by activation of membrane bounded GC which is regulated by peptides including the natriuretic peptides (see Tremblay et al.,1988). In the periphery, morphine may exert its analgesic effect via activation of soluble GC. Centrally, activation of the GC system may be direct via direct stimulation of membrane GC, without NO intermediation. In addition to this mechanism, morphine may also block activation of adenylate cyclase or activate GC . This double mechanism may explain the high central analgesic potency of morphine. It is not yet understood the contribution for neuronal excitability the chain of biochemical events that follows either the blockade of adenylate cyclase activation nor the stimulation of GC activation. It should be pointed out that tolerance occurs only for the central but not for the peripheral action of morphine (Ferreira et al., 1984). It is intriguing that the molecular events that follows morphine central and peripheral receptor activation are probably different. Centrally, is dependent of a double receptor mediated mechanism, blockade of adenylate cyclase activation and stimulation of membrane GC. In the periphery, however, the mechanism of morphine is indirect, due to soluble GC activation, via the release of NO. Negative modulation of adenilatecyclase activity, changes in Ca^{2+} and neuronal membrane composition have been evoked in attempts to establish a possible causal relationship between opiate stimulation and the analgesic effect (for review, see Ronai and Székely, 1982). However none of them was demonstrated to be correlated with the mechanism of analgesic action of morphine. The experiments described in this study are the first demonstration that links peripheral and central analgesic effect of morphine to the stimulation of GC system. Those effects of morphine upon adenilate and GC systems, may explain the enormous variety of metabolic effects of opiates.

REFERENCES :

Azami, J.; Llewelyn, M.B. and Roberts, M.H.T. The contribution of Nucleus Reticularis Paragigantocellularis and Nucleus Raphe Magnus to the analgesia produced by systemically administered morphine, investigated with microinjection technique. Pain 12, 229-246 (1982).

Ferreira, S.H. Prostaglandins, peripheral and central analgesia. In Advances in Pain Research and Therapy vol.5 (eds Bonica, J.J.) 627-634 (Raven Press, New York), 1983.

Ferreira, S.H. and Nakamura, M. I- Prosrtaglandin hyperalgesia: A cAMP/Ca++ dependent process. Prostaglandins 18, 179-190 (1979).

Ferreira, S.H.; Lorenzetti, B.B. and Correa, F.M.A. Central and peripheral antialgic action of aspirin-like drugs. European J. Pharmacol. 53, 39 (1978).

Ferreira, S.H.; Lorenzetti, B.B. and Rae, G.A. European J. Pharmacol. 99, 23-9 (1984).

Lorenzetti, B.B. and Ferreira, S.H. On the mode of analgesic action of Tyr-D-arg-Gly-Phe [4-NO2] Pro-NH (443c). Br.J.Pharmacol. 90, 68p (1987).

Moncada, S.; Palmer, R.M.J. and Higgs, E.A. The discovery of nitric oxide as the endogenous nitrovasodilator. Hypertension 12, 365-72 (1988).

Palmer, R.M.J.; Ashton, D.S and Moncada,S. Vascular endothelial cells sinthetize nitric oxide from L-arginine. Nature 33, 664 (1988a)

Palmer, R.M.J.; Rees, D.D. and Moncada, S. L-arginine is the physiological precursor for formation of nitric oxide in the endothelium-dependent relaxation. Bioch. Biophys. Res. Comm. 153, 1251 (1988b).

Rees, D.D.; Palmer, R.M.J.; Hodson, F. and Moncada, S. Specific inhibitor of nitric oxide formation from L-arginine attenuates endothelium-dependent relaxation. Br. J. Pharmacol. 96, 418-24 (1989).

Ronai, A.Z. and Székely, J.I. In: Opioides Peptides vol.2 (eds Székely, J.I.) 1-32 (CRF Press, Bocaraton, 1982).

Tremblay, J., Gerzer, R. and Hamet, P. Cyclic GMP in cells function. Advances in second messenger and phosphoprotein Res. 22, 319-383 (1988).

AAS 32
Drugs in Inflammation

PROSTAGLANDIN (PG) MODULATION OF BRADYKININ-INDUCED HYPERALGESIA AND OEDEMA IN THE GUINEA-PIG PAW - EFFECTS OF PGD_2, PGE_2 AND PGI_2

C.J. Whelan, S.A. Head, C.T. Poll† and R.A. Coleman

Department of Peripheral Pharmacology, Glaxo Group Research Ltd., Ware, Herts., U.K.

† present address: Preclinical Pharmacology, Sandoz Ltd., CH-4002, Basle, Switzerland.

SUMMARY: The relative potencies of PGD_2, PGE_2 and PGI_2 in potentiating bradykinin-induced hyperalgesia and oedema were determined in the paws of aspirin-treated guinea-pigs. PGE_2 and to a lesser degree PGD_2 but not PGI_2, potentiated bradykinin-induced hyperalgesia, whereas PGD_2, but not PGE_2 or PGI_2, potentiated oedema. These findings differ from those in other species, and possibly reflect interspecies differences in modulation of inflammatory reactions by prostanoids.

INTRODUCTION

Hyperalgesia and oedema are two features of the acute inflammatory response which are modulated by prostanoids (see Vane, 1976; Ferreira, 1981). Studies in rats have indicated that prostacyclin appears to play a role in inflammatory pain and oedema (Ferreira et al., 1978; Ford-Hutchinson et al., 1978; Higgs et al., 1978). The present report describes experiments designed to determine the relative potencies of some natural prostanoids in potentiating bradykinin (BK)-induced hyperalgesia and oedema in the guinea-pig paw.

METHODS

Female guinea-pigs of body weight 150-200g were used. All animals were pretreated with aspirin (200mg/kg i.p.) to inhibit endogenous prostanoid synthesis. Thirty minutes after aspirin treatment, the resting nociceptive pressure threshold (NPT) for the left hind paw of each guinea-pig was determined using an analgesymeter (Ugo Basile, Milan). The NPT was then measured again thirty minutes later. At the same time, the volume of the right hind paw was measured by immersing the paw in a plethysmometer (Ugo Basile, Milan) to a line drawn around the tarsus. Each guinea-pig was then given a sub-plantar injection into the right hind paw of vehicle, bradykinin, the prostaglandin under test or combinations of BK and prostaglandin, in 100µl of sterile saline. Right hind paw volume (PV) and NPT were then determined at intervals. The operator of the analgesymeter was unaware of the treatment assigned to each animal.

Data are expressed as increases in PV (%) and decreases in NPT (analgesymeter units) from pre-injection values.

Drugs and reagents: Aspirin (Sigma) was dissolved in sodium bicarbonate such that a volume of 1.0ml/kg was administered i.p. PGE_2 (Upjohn) and PGD_2 (Glaxo Group Research) were dissolved in 3% ethanol/0.01% Tween 80 in sterile saline to a stock concentration of 10^{-3}mol/l. Dilutions were made in sterile saline. Prostacyclin (PGI_2; Glaxo Group Research) was dissolved in tris buffer (pH 9.0) at a concentration of 10^{-3}mol/l and further diluted in tris buffer (pH 8.0) immediately prior to use.

RESULTS

Preliminary experiments demonstrated that NPT in the left hind paw was comparable to that in the right hind paw of the guinea-pigs, and therefore this was used as the control value for all determinations. In aspirin-pretreated guinea-pigs, subplantar injection of BK (10^{-8}mol/paw) caused an immediate vocalisation which was transient (≈1min). Following this initial response, BK had little effect on NPT but caused a small, transient increase in PV (27.0 ± 6.0%, n=6) 1-2h after injection.

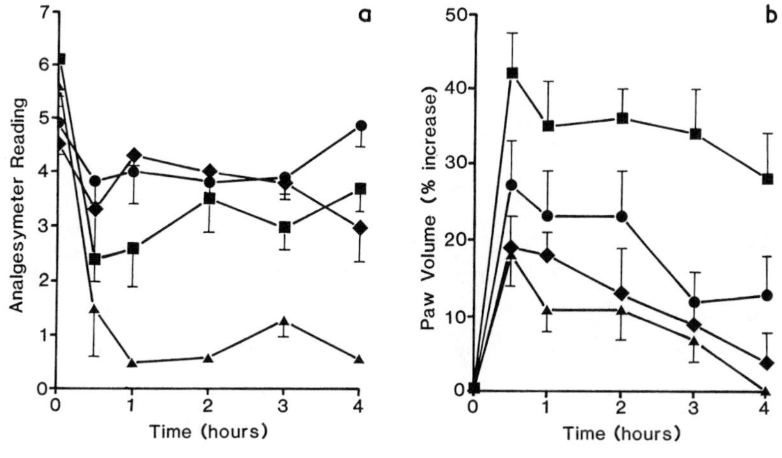

Figure 1: Hyperalgesia (left panel) and increase in paw volume (right panel) in aspirin-treated guinea-pigs in response to bradykinin (10^{-8}mol/paw) alone (●), and in combination with 10^{-7}mol/paw PGD_2 (■), PGE_2 (▲) or PGI_2 (♦).

PGE_2 (10^{-7}mol/paw) alone caused a significant decrease in NPT ($P<0.05$) from a control value of 5.9 ± 0.4 to 2.7 ± 0.9 (n=6). This decrease developed 60 min after injection, and then remained constant for the rest of the experiment. Neither PGD_2 nor PGI_2 (10^{-7}mol/paw) alone had any significant effect on NPT. PGE_2 and PGD_2 (10^{-7}mol/paw) both caused small apparent increases in PV. However, these increases in PV were variable in degree, and not statistically significant when compared with control (vehicle) values ($p>0.05$, Student's t-test). PGI_2 (10^{-7}mol/paw) had no obvious effect on PV.

When co-administered with BK (10^{-8}mol/paw), PGE_2 (10^{-7}mol/paw) caused an immediate marked decrease in NPT from 5.6 ± 0.4 to 0.5 ± 0 (n=6) which persisted for the duration (4h) of the experiment (Fig 1). PGE_2 also caused a small transient increase in PV (18 ± 4%, n=6), which was evident 30 min after injection. In contrast, co-administration of PGD_2 (10^{-7}mol/paw, n=6) with BK caused a smaller decrease in NPT from 6.1 ± 0.7 to 2.4 ± 0.4 (Fig 1), but a marked, persistent increase in PV (42.0 ± 6.0%). Co-administration of PGI_2 with BK had no significant effect ($p>0.05$) on NPT or PV over that produced by BK alone (Fig 1).

DISCUSSION

These results show that in guinea-pig paw, neither PGE_2, PGD_2 or PGI_2 when administered alone has any marked proinflammatory activity, However, PGE_2, and to a lesser degree PGD_2, but not PGI_2, appears to modulate BK-induced hyperalgesia; whereas PGD_2, but not PGE_2 or PGI_2, enhances BK-induced oedema. These findings contrast with those reported from experiments in rats, where PGI_2 is more potent than PGE_2 in inducing both hyperalgesia and oedema (Ferreira et al., 1978; Ford-Hutchinson et al., 1978; Higgs et al., 1978). This difference in the relative effects of the prostanoids in guinea-pigs and rats is unlikely to be due to the removal of endogenous prostanoids by cyclooxygenase inhibition, since the experiments of Ferreira et al. (1978) and Higgs et al. (1978) were also conducted in indomethacin-pretreated animals. A more likely explanation is that it reflects species differences in response to prostanoids. In conclusion, the experiments described above demonstrate that in guinea-pig paw, PGE_2 modulates BK-induced hyperalgesia, whereas PGD_2 modulates BK-induced oedema. We suggest that the differences between our findings and those reported by others reflect differences in the prostanoid receptors modulating aspects of the inflammatory response in these different species. If, indeed, this is the case, similar data from clinical studies are essential in order to determine which species most closely mimics responses in man.

REFERENCES

Ferreira, S.H. (1981). Inflammatory pain, prostaglandin hyperalgesia and the development of peripheral analgesics. T.I.P.S. vol 2, pp 183-186.

Ferreira, S.H., Nakamura, M., Castro, M.S.A. (1978). The hyperalgesic effects of prostacyclin and prostaglandin E_2. Prostaglandins, vol 16, pp 31-37.

Ford-Hutchinson, A.W., Walker, J.R., Davidson, E.M., Smith, M.J.H. (1978). PGI_2: A potential mediator of inflammation. Prostaglandins, vol 16 pp 253-258.

Higgs, E.A., Moncada, S., Vane, J.R. (1978). Inflammatory effects of prostacyclin (PGI_2) and 6-oxo-$PGF_{1\alpha}$ in the rat paw. Prostaglandins, vol 16, pp 153-162.

Vane, J.R. (1976). The mode of action of aspirin and similar compounds. J. Allergy Clin. Immunol., vol 58, pp 691-712.

AAS 32
Drugs in Inflammation

ANALGETIC ACTIVITY OF SK&F 105809, A DUAL INHIBITOR OF ARACHIDONIC ACID METABOLISM.

D.E. Griswold, P. Marshall, L. Martin, E.F. Webb, and B. Zabko-Potapovich.

Division of Pharmacological Sciences, SmithKline Beecham Pharmaceuticals
P.O. Box 1539, King of Prussia, PA, U.S.A.

SUMMARY: The analgetic activity of inhibitors of 5-lipoxygenase (5-LO) and cyclooxygenase (CO) was investigated using rat Randall-Selitto (RS) hyperalgesia and mouse phenylbenzoquinone (PBQ)-induced abdominal constriction assays. Using the RS assay, the CO inhibitors indomethacin, naproxen, and ibuprofen all effectively reduced hyperalgesia; whereas, the inhibitors of leukotriene production, MK886 and phenidone were inactive. SK&F 105809, a dual inhibitor of 5-LO/CO, significantly reduced hyperalgesia. In the PBQ assay, CO inhibitors were active, SK&F 105809 was nearly as potent as naproxen, and MK886 and phenidone were found to be active. Thus, improved analgetic activity appeared to result from inhibition of 5-LO and CO; whereas, in the RS assay, only CO inhibitors and SK&F 105809 were clearly effective. These results suggest that dual inhibitors, and in particular, SK&F 105809 may be more efficient analgesic agents than selective CO inhibitors in clinical situations in which 5-LO products play a signficant role.

INTRODUCTION

Analgesia is a clinically beneficial property of non steroidal antiinflammatory drugs (NSAID). This property has been associated with selective cyclooxygenase inhibitors where a correlation between inhibition of cyclooxygenase and analgetic potency in animal models and clinical activity in man has been seen (Doherty, 1987; Lewis et al., 1983). Although it has been suggested that lipoxygenase products are hyperalgesic (Levine et al., 1984), the impact of *in vivo* inhibition of lipoxygenase products on analgetic potency is still unknown. Therefore, it was of interest to determine the analgetic activity and potency of SK&F 105809 since it is an inhibitor of both the cyclooxygenase and lipoxygenase pathways of arachidonic acid metabolism (Hanna et al., 1990). This was done using the standard assays: Randall-Selitto induced hyperalgesia and phenylbenzoquinone-induced algesia. Both assays have been widely used to evaluate NSAID analgesia and have also been suggested to have a lipoxygenase component (Opas, et al., 1987; Carey et al., 1988).

METHODS AND MATERIALS

Animals: Female CD outbred Sprague Dawley rats (80-100g) and male CD1 mice (25-42) were obtained from Charles River Breeding Laboratories (Kingston, NY). Three to six animals were used per group.

Compounds and Reagents: SK&F 105809 was synthesized by K. Erhard and MK-886 was obtained from the Drug Substances and Products Registry of SmithKline Beecham. SK&F 105809 was dissolved in acidified saline and was administered orally. Naproxen, ibuprofen, indomethacin, and phenidone were purchased from Sigma Chemical Co., St. Louis, MO, were suspended in 0.5% tragacanth and administered orally. Phenylbenzoquinone (PBQ, Eastman Kodak Co., Rochester, NY.) was dissolved in 50°C ethanol, diluted with distilled water to a final concentration of 0.2 mg/ml, and administered intraperitoneally. The dose volume for all compounds was 0.01 ml/gm.

Randall-Selitto Assay (RS): An injection of 0.1 ml of a 20% brewer's yeast-water suspension was placed into the right hind paw of the rat at 0 time. At 1.5 hours post yeast injection the rats were treated orally with compound or vehicle. At 2.5 hours post yeast injection the pain threshold of the rat's injected paw was measured by a pressure device (Analgesia-Meter, Ugo Basile,Italy). The endpoint was measured in grams of force necessary to elicit paw withdrawal.

Phenylquinone-induced abdominal constriction Assay (PBQ): Mice were pre-treated with vehicle or test compound 15 mins and following PBQ injection, each mouse was placed into individual 4 liter beakers. Abdominal constriction or stretching responses were counted on a hand counter. The counting period was for 10 mins following a 5 min acclimation period.

Data Analysis and Statistics: Mean values for groups were calculated and percent inhibition was determined between the vehicle control mean and test group. The ED50 was determined using linear regression analysis. Statistical analysis was done using Student's "t" test and a $p < 0.05$ was considered statistically significant.

RESULTS

Effect of CO and 5-LO inhibition on RS Hyperalgesia: The analgetic activity of the CO inhibitors, indomethacin, naproxen and ibuprofen; the 5-LO inhibitor phenidone and 5-LO translocation inhibitor MK-886; and the dual inhibitor SK&F 105809 as determined in dose response experiments. As seen in Table I, the CO inhibitors were potent analgetic agents and their potency agreed reasonably well with their reported CO inhibitory activity. In contrast, the 5-LO translocation inhibitor, MK-886 and the lipoxygenase inhibitor phenidone were without significant effect at doses inhibitory to LTB_4 production, while the dual inhibitor, SK&F 105809 had significant activity.

Table I. Effect of CO,5-LO and Dual Inhibitors on RS Hyperalgesia

Compound	ED50, mg/kg, p.o.
Indomethacin	9
Naproxen	14
Ibuprofen	37
Phenidone	>200
MK-886	>10
SK&F 105809	86

Phenylquinone-induced algesia: Likewise, CO inhibitors were found to be active in PBQ assay and the rank-order compared well with their CO inhibition. In contrast to RS assay, MK886 and phenidone were active (Table II). SK&F 105809 showed improved activity and inhibited the response to PBQ with a potency comparable to naproxen (ED50 19 vs 9 mg/kg, p.o., respectively).

Table II. Effect of CO, 5-LO, and Dual Inhibitors on PBQ Algesia.

Compound	ED50 mg/kg, p.o.
Indomethacin	0.6
Naproxen	9.4
Ibuprofen	14.7
Phenidone	50 (~ED35)
MK-886	4.9 (ED25)
SK&F 105809	19

DISCUSSION

The results of this evaluation indicated that SK&F 105809 had analgetic activity as shown by the RS and PBQ-induced abdominal constriction assay. These assays are generally considered to detect the analgetic activity of cyclooxygenase inhibitors thus their activity was expected. However, it was surprising to find that SK&F 105809, which has considerably less cyclooxygenase inhibitory activity than naproxen (Hanna et al., 1990), exhibited only slightly lower analgesic activity, suggesting that additional factors contributed to the potency of SK&F 105809. Since SK&F 150809 is a dual inhibitor of both cyclooxygenase and lipoxygenase, it follows that synergy between these two activities may provide this compound with superior analgetic activity as compared to selective cyclooxygenase inhibitors. In support of this suggestion is the observation that LTB_4 causes hyperalgesia (Levine et al., 1984). In the case of the RS assay, other factors may contribute since compounds which inhibit 5-LO product formation are inactive.

The analgetic effect of SK&F 105809 appears not to be mediated through opioid receptors since naloxone did not antagonize its activity in the PBQ assay (data not shown). In conclusion, these results suggest that SK&F 105809 may have utility in the treatment of inflammatory pain.

Acknowledgements: The authors are grateful to Dr. Nabil Hanna for his guidance and support.

REFERENCES

Carey, F., Haworth, D., Edmonds, A.E., and Forder, R.A. (1988) Simple Procedure for Measuring the Pharmacodynamics and Analgeic Potential of Lipoxygenase Inhibitors. J. Pharm. Methods. 20, 347-356.

Doherty, N.S. (1987) Mediators of the Pain of Inflammation. Annual Reports in Med. Chem. 22,245-252.

Hanna, N., Marshall, P.J., Newton, J. Jr., Schwartz, L., Kirsh, R., DiMartino, M.J., Adams, J., Bender, P. and Griswold, D.E.(1990) Pharmacological profile of SK&F 105809, a dual inhibitor of arachidonic acid metabolism. Drugs Under Experimental and Clinical Research (In Press).

Levine, J.D., W. Lau, and G. Kwait (1984) Leukotriene B_4 produces hyperalgesia that is dependent upon polymorphonuclear leukocytes. Science. 225, 743-745.

Lewis, A.J., Carlson, R.P., Chang. J., Gilman, S.C., Nielsen, S., Rosenthale, M.E., Janssen, F.W. and Ruelius, H.W. (1983) The Pharmacological Profile of Oxaprozin, an Antiinflammatory and Analgesic Agent with Low Gastrointestinal Toxicity. Current Therapeutic Res. 34, 777-794.

Opas, E.E., Dallob, A., Herold, E., Luell, S., and Humes, J.L. (1987) Pharmacological Modulation of Eicosanoid levels and Hyperalgesia in Yeast-induced Inflammation. Biochem. Pharm. 36, 547-551.

AAS 32
Drugs in Inflammation

PHARMACOLOGICAL PROFILE OF FLUPIRTINE, A NOVEL CENTRALLY ACTING, NON-OPIOD ANALGESIC DRUG

I. Szelenyi and B. Nickel

Department of Pharmacology, ASTA Pharma AG, POB 100105, 6000 Frankfurt /M. 1, FRG

SUMMARY: Flupirtine is a new non-opioid, non-addicting centrally acting analgesic. In animals, antinociceptive activity of flupirtine was attenuated after reserpine pretreatment or in the presence of α-adrenergic antagonists suggesting the possible involvement of the noradrenergic system in its analgesic mode of action. Additionally, flupirtine possesses skeletal muscle relaxing activity in rats.

INTRODUCTION

Flupirtine, a novel, non-opioid, non-addicting, centrally acting analgesic compound has recently been introduced in the therapy of painful disorders. It has been demonstrated that its peripheral analgesic activity is low, when compared to that of non-steroidal anti-inflammatory drugs (Jakovlev et al., 1985). Previous observations clearly indicate that flupirtine acts to produce its effects through a central action in which opioid or benzodiazepine mechanisms are not involved, at all (Carlsson and Jurna, 1988; Nickel et al., 1985, 1990). Recent data suggest that flupirtine presumably needs the noradrenergic system to elicit its antinociceptive action (Szelenyi and Nickel,1987; Szelenyi et al., 1989). In the present paper, we demonstrate some results obtained with flupirtine and focuss the interest on an additional effect of this analagesic observed recently in animal experiments.

MATERIALS AND METHODS

Animals: Sprague-Dawley (SIV 50) rats (190-220g) or mice (NMRI) (20-25g) (Fa.Savo, Kisslegg, FRG) were used. Animals were maintained under standard environmental conditions (room temperature: 21-22°C; relative humidity: 55-60%; light-dark-rhythm: 12/12h). They had free access to standard pellet food and drinking water but 18 h before the experiments they were deprived of food.

Tail-flick test: Ten min after intraperitoneal administration of flupirtine the antinociceptive action was evaluated by the tail flick test using an automated unit (Hugo Sachs Electronic, Hugstetten,FRG). The intensity of the light beam was adjusted so that base-line readings were generally at about 5-6 s, and a 20 s cut-off was imposed to avoid excessive tissue damage.

Electrostimulated pain: 30 min after oral administration of flupirtine the animals were placed on a metal screen and stimulated with increasing square-wave current until they reacted with vocalization showing the pain threshold. Analgesic activity was expressed as a percentage increase in the pain threshold in comparison to the control animals. Prazosin, idazoxane and reserpine were administered intraperitoneally at appropriate times prior to flupirtine.

Measurement of muscle tone: The measurement of the muscle rigidity was performed by recording successively the resistance of flexors and extensors which counteracted the forced straightening and bending of the foot in the ankle joint. During the measurement the rat was placed in a special well-ventilated cage. The hind limb foot, protruding from a special opening in the bottom of the cage, was slipped into an appropriately matched box (rat shoe). The axis, allowing rotations of the rat shoe, was placed exactly under the ankle joint. The localization of the axis stabilized the position of foot and allowed the measurement of the response restricted to flexors or extensors of the foot. Furthermore, a rigid steel rod was sunk into the base of the box and the other side was inserted into a measurement opening of a force sensor. So each change in the pressure exerted by the the foot on the box was measured immediately by the force transducer.

RESULTS

The pretreatment of mice with the storage depleting compound, reserpine, almost totally abolished the antinociceptive effect of flupirtine in the electrostimulated test. In the presence of idazoxane and prazosin, the analgesic activity of flupirtine has been attenuated (Table 1).

Table.1. Effect of pretreatment with reserpine, prazosin and idazoxane on the antinociceptive activity of oral flupirtine in mice using electrostimulated pain test

	increase in pain threshold (%)
Flupirtine 20 mg/kg p.o.	62 %
+ reserpine 2 mg/kg i.p.	8 %
+ prazosin 2 mg/kg i.p.	3 %
+ idazoxane 2 mg/kg i.p.	5 %

Prazosin, idazoxane and reserpine were given intraperitoneally 0.5, 0.5 and 18 hours prior to flupirtine administration

Reserpine-induced muscle rigidity has been inhibited dose-dependently by flupirtine. The ED_{50}- value amounted to 5.6 mg/kg i.p. which is closely related to the antinociceptive ED_{50}-value established in the tail-flick test (7.8 mg/kg, i.p.). Diazepam reduced reserpine-induced muscle rigidity by 50% at the dose of 5.2 mg/kg i.p.

DISCUSSION

Flupirtine has been demonstrated to be a centrally acting analgesic. Its mode of antinociceptive action is clearly different from that of opioids. Based on previous results, it is unlikely that the antinociceptive action of flupirtine is mediated via serotonergic descending pathways (Szelenyi et al.,1989). With regard to our former and present results, it is likely that the noradrenergic system in the central nervous system could be involved in the antinociceptive mode of action of flupirtine. Further investigation, however, is needed to confirm or disprove this working hypothesis.

The most important finding of the present work is that flupirtine is able to abolish the reserpine-induced rigidity of the skeletal muscle in rats in a dose-range closely related to its antinociceptive activity.The presice mode of the muscle relaxing action of flupirtine is not known. Until now, no analgesic compound with a skeletal muscle relaxing activity is known. Therefore, this additional property of flupirtine may be of significance in the treatment of disorders accompained by muscle tenseness.

REFERENCES

Carlsson, K.-H. and I. Jurna (1987) Depression by flupirtine, a novel analgesic agent, of motor and sensory responses of the nociceptive system in the rat spinal cord, Eur. J. Pharmacol. 143,89-99.

Jakovlev, V., Sofia, R.D., Achterrath-Tuckermann, U., von Schlichtegroll, A. and Thiemer, K. (1985) Untersuchungen zur pharmakologischen Wirkung von Flupirtin, einem strukturell neuartigen Analgetikum, Arzneim.-Forsch./Drug Res.,35,30-34.

Nickel, B., H.O. Borbe and Szelenyi I. (1990) Flupirtine has no benzodiazepine - like abuse potential, Arzneim.-Forsch./Drug Res. in press

Nickel, B., Engel, J. and Szelenyi, I. (1988) Possible involvement of noradrenergic descending painmodulating pathways in the mode of antinociceptive action of flupirtine, a novel non-opioid analgesic, Agents Actions 23,112-116.

Nickel, B., Herz, A., Jakovlev, V. and Tibes, U. (1985) Untersuchungen zum Wirkungsmechanismus des Analgetikums Flupirtin, Arzneim.-Forsch./Drug Res. 35, 1402-1405.

Szelenyi, I. and B. Nickel (1987) Putative site(s) and mechanism(s) of flupirtine, a novel analgesic compound, Postgrad. Med. J. 63 (Suppl.3), 57-60.

Szelenyi, I., B. Nickel, H.O. Borbe and K. Brune (1989) Mode of antinociceptive action of flupirtine in the rats, Br. J. Pharmacol. 97, 835-842.

AAS 32
Drugs in Inflammation

THE PHARMACOLOGICAL PROFILE OF ACECLOFENAC, A NEW NONSTEROIDAL ANTIINFLAMMATORY AND ANALGESIC DRUG

M. Grau, J.L. Montero, J. Guasch, A. Felipe, E. Carrasco and S. Juliá

Department of Pharmacology and Toxicology, Prodesfarma Research Center, Trabajo s/n, 08960, Sant Just Desvern (Barcelona, Spain)

SUMMARY: Aceclofenac is a new phenylacetic acid derivative provided with marked antiinflammatory, antiarthritic, analgesic and antipyretic activities in animal experimental models. While maintaining its potency Aceclofenac demonstrates better gastric tolerance and consequently offers greater potential security than other highly active agents such as Indomethacin and Diclofenac.

INTRODUCTION

Nonsteroidal antiinflammatory drugs (NSAIDs) are widely used in the treatment of a number of arthritic conditions, but gastrointestinal lesions have often limited their clinical utilization. To obtain newer potent NSAIDs with improved gastrointestinal tolerability, we have synthesized and screened a series of phenylacetic acid derivatives. Among them 2-[(2,6-dichlorophenyl) amine] phenylacetoxiacetic acid (Aceclofenac, ACF) showed good antiinflammatory activity and weak gastric irritative effects when assayed in rats, and hence it was selected for further study. Therapeutic efficacy and tolerance of ACF has been demonstrated in Phase I and Phase II clinical trials and this drug is now undergoing extensive Phase III multicentric studies. In this paper, the pharmacological profile of ACF is compared to that of Indomethacin (IND), Diclofenac (DICL), Naproxen (NAP) and Phenylbutazone (PBZ).

MATERIAL AND METHODS

Acute inflammatory models: The effects of ACF and reference drugs on carrageenin-induced paw edema (Winter et al., 1962), carrageenin-induced abscess (Benitz & Hall, 1963) and carrageenin-induced pleurisy (Vinegar et al., 1981) were examined in Sprague Dawley and Wistar male rats. The inhibitory effect on increased vascular permeability (Whittle, 1964) was evaluated in Swiss male mice. Beagle dogs were used in the sodium urate crystal-induced synovitis model (Niemegeers & Janssen, 1975).

Chronic inflammatory models: Cotton pellet-induced granuloma (Winter & Porter, 1957) and adjuvant-induced arthritis (Pearson, 1965) were performed in male and female SD rats respectively, according to standard methodologies with slight modifications. Arthritis was produced by intraplantar injection into the right paw of a suspension of *Mycobacterium butyricum* in mineral oil. Tested compounds were given orally once daily for 21 consecutive days in prophylactic experiments, and from 14 to 28 days after *M. butyricum* in therapeutic assays.

Analgesic effects: To test antihyperalgesic activity phenylquinone-induced writhing in mice, compression of yeast-inflamed paw in rats, and flection pain in silver nitrate-induced arthralgia in rats were used (Kameyama et al., 1987).

Antipyretic effect: Yeast-induced febrile male SD rats were used to evaluate antipyretic actions (Rouveix, 1980).

Gastric ulcerogenic effects: Gastric ulceration induced by ACF and reference drugs was examined in fasted male Wistar rats after single oral dosing. The animals were killed 6h after the administration of drugs and the degree of gastric lesions was then evaluated macroscopically according to Lwoff (1971).

Acute toxicity: Mortality and symptoms were evaluated in male Wistar rats within 15 days after oral dosing with tested drugs.

RESULTS AND DISCUSSION

ACF has been shown to be highly effective in the acute inflammatory models, with a potency comparable to that of IND and DICL and better than that of NAP and PBZ (Table I). Oral administration of ACF (0.6-5.4 mg/kg) prior to intraarticular injection of sodium urate in dogs also improved dose-dependently the animals' impaired gait (Table I). ACF given orally (2.5-10 mg/kg/day) for seven consecutive days inhibited the granuloma formation in the rat cotton pellet test, with a maximum value of 32% at the highest dose assayed (Table I). In chronic test of adjuvant-induced arthritis in rats ACF administered both in prophylactic and therapeutic regimens (0.5-2 mg/kg/day, p.o.), displayed good antiarthritic activity against primary and secondary inflammatory responses, being equipotent to IND and DICL. Notable analgesic activity was demonstrated for ACF in a number of animal models of pain elicited by chemical, mechanical or arthritic algic stimuli, with a potency comparable to that

Table I. Antiinflammatory effects of ACF and reference drugs in several models of acute and chronic inflammation.

Test	Drugs				
	ACF	IND	DICL	NAP	PBZ
Effective doses (mg/kg, p.o.):					
Anti-edema[a]	3.59	2.21	3.93	8.11	32.13
Anti-abscess[b]	1.10	1.55	1.45	2.72	12.02
Anti-pleurisy[b,d]	10.21	2.92	11.00	4.14	48.17
Vascular permeability[a]	7.79	3.01	3.54	17.13	93.95
Urate synovitis[a]	1.20	--	--	--	--
Anti-granuloma[c]	4.63	3.55	7.19	24.43	121.66

a) ED_{50} b) ED_{30} c) ED_{25} d) Suppression of the pleural effusive response.

Table II. Analgesic and antipyretic effects of ACF and reference drugs in rodents.

Test	Drugs ACF	IND	DICL	NAP	PBZ
ED_{50} (mg/kg, p.o.):					
Phenylquinone writhing	3.28	1.04	4.26	14.36	47.05
Randall and Selitto	0.76	1.85	1.00	8.54	38.63
Silver nitrate flection	0.79	3.97	1.11	4.47	92.02
Yeast-induced fever	0.43	3.01	0.18	1.86	22.10

of DICL and IND (Table II). Like other NSAIDs, ACF has a predominant peripheral mechanism of analgesic action. ACF also reduced hyperthermia in brewer's yeast-febrile rats in a dose-dependent manner (Table II). However, the most striking pharmacological feature of ACF is its lower gastric ulcerogenic activity under acute test conditions, if compared to the most active reference NSAIDs tested (Table III). So, ACF is 4-7 times weaker than IND and DICL in terms of number of animals damaged and severity of lesions. This fact is also reflected in its lower acute toxicity (Table III). Hence, safety coefficients of ACF were 1.5-4 times higher than those of reference NSAIDs.

Table III. Gastric ulcerogenic effects, acute toxicity and safety coefficients for ACF and reference drugs in rats.

Test	Drugs ACF	IND	DICL	NAP	PBZ
Gastric ulceration (UD50 mg/kg, p.o.)	24.32	3.57	6.22	14.86	142.81
Acute toxicity (LD50 mg/kg, p.o.)	129.76	20.32	68.59	247.46	636.93
Safety coefficients:					
1) UD50/ED50*	6.8	1.6	1.6	1.8	4.4
2) LD50/ED50*	36.1	9.2	17.4	30.5	19.8

*Antiinflammatory activity in the carrageenin-induced paw edema in rats.

CONCLUSIONS

In summary, ACF maintains good antiinflammatory and analgesic potency in animal models, while it has lower gastric toxicity after acute administration than other highly active representative NSAIDs such as IND and DICL.

REFERENCES

Benitz, K.F., and Hall, L.M. (1963) The carrageenin-induced abscess as a new test for antiinflammatory activity of steroids and nonsteroids. Arch. int. Pharmacodyn. 144, 185-195.

Kameyama, T., Nabeshima, T., Yamada, S., and Sato, M. (1987) Analgesic and antiinflammatory effects of CN-100 in rat and mouse. Arzneim. Forsch. 37(1), 19-26.

Lwoff, J.M. (1971) Ulcerogenic activity test in rats. J. Pharmacol. (Paris) 2(1), 81-83.

Niemegeers, C.J.E., and Janssen, P.A.J. (1975) Suprofen, a potent antagonist of sodium urate crystal-induced arthritis in dogs. Arzneim. Forsch. 25(10), 1512-1515.

Rouveix, B. (1980) Brewer's yeast-induced hyperthermia test in rats. J. Pharmacol. (Paris) 11(1), 133-136.

Pearson, C.M. (1965) Development of arthritis, periarthitis and periostitis in rats given adjuvant. P.S.E.B.M. 91, 95-100.

Vinegar, R., Truax, J.F., Selph, J.L., Johnston, P.R., Venable, A.L., and Voelker, F.A. (1981) Development of carrageenan pleurisy in the rat: effects of colchicine on inhibition of cell mobilization. Ibid. 168, 24-32.

Whittle, B.A. (1964) The use of changes in capillary permeability in mice to distinguish between narcotic and nonnarcotic analgesics. Brit. J. Pharmacol. 22, 246-253.

Winter, C.A., and Porter C.C. (1957) Effect of alterations in side chain upon antiinflammatory and liver glycogen activities of hydrocortisone esters. J. Amer. Pharmac. Assoc. 46(9), 515-519.

Winter, C.A., Risley, E.A., and Nuss, G.W. (1962) Carrageenin-induced edema in hind paw of the rat as an assay for antiinflammatory drugs. P.S.E.B.M. 111, 544-547.

New Treatments for Bone and Cartilage Loss in Rheumatoid Arthritis

AAS 32
Drugs in Inflammation

MOLECULAR BASIS OF INTRACELLULAR INTERACTIONS IN RELATION TO BONE AND JOINT DISEASE

R.G.G. Russell

Department of Human Metabolism and Clinical Biochemistry
University of Sheffield Medical School, Beech Hill Rd
Sheffield S10 2RX, UK

SUMMARY

During the past 10 years there have been impressive advances in knowledge about regulatory mechanisms that may be involved in connective tissue turnover in health and disease. It is now generally accepted that cells within the tissues of bone and joints are responsive to a wide variety of agents, many of which may act in an autocrine or paracrine manner. We will review the role of systemic hormones and locally active factors in the regulation of bone metabolism and on the activity of chondrocytes, synovial cells, and on cells in the immune system in relation to joint disease. The biochemical basis of these processes will be reviewed with particular emphasis on the roles of interleukin-1, tumour necrosis factor, the interferons, as well as other cytokines and growth factors. Such factors can account for many of the systemic manifestations of chronic inflammatory disease, as well as the local degradation and repair processes within connective tissues. The therapeutic effects of drugs such as glucocorticoids and cyclosporin A may be partly explicable in terms of their intervention with these regulatory mechanisms. The rapid rate of increase in knowledge about these biochemical processes offers great potential for the future understanding of the pathogenic mechanisms involved in disease processes affecting skeletal tissues. It also offers hope of finding ways of creating new drugs that intervene effectively in these processes.

AAS 32
Drugs in Inflammation

THE ROLE OF PROTEINASES IN CARTILAGE DESTRUCTION

C. H. Evans

Department of Biochemistry and Cell Biology, Hunterian Institute, Royal College of Surgeons of England, London, WC2A 3PN, England.

SUMMARY: Most of the organic, extracellular matrix of articular cartilage consists of collagens and proteoglycans. Their degradation is initiated extra- or peri-cellularly by proteinases produced locally by cells in and around the joint. Although enzymes from all four classes of proteinases can degrade the cartilagenous matrix, serine proteinases, particularly plasmin, and various neutral metalloproteinases (NMPs) are likely to be the key enzymes in this process. Much attention has been paid to members of the latter group, which are synthesised both by the resident, mesenchymal cells of the joint and by various types of white blood cells which colonise it during inflammation. NMPs can be conveniently grouped into three classes, the collagenases, the stromelysins and the gelatinases. Two members are known for each class, with the recently identified "pump" (Putative Metalloproteinase) probably constituting a third member of the stromelysin group. Regulation of these enzymes is complex. Cells normally synthesise NMPs at low rates, but their production increases markedly following cellular activation by cytokines or certain other stimuli. Major control points for enzyme synthesis occur at the levels of transcription and the conversion of proenzyme to active enzyme; enzyme activity is further regulated through the action of inhibitors. Alpha-2 macroglobulin is the major systemic inhibitor, while a number of tissue inhibitors act as local regulators. These include at least two TIMPs and several IMPs. Pharmacologic manipulation of NMP activity holds promise as an approach to anti-erosive therapy in arthritis.

INTRODUCTION: Although the various components of the cartilaginous matrix are degraded during normal metabolic turnover, it is the exaggerated breakdown occurring in arthritis that has attracted most experimental attention. In quantitative terms, the destruction of articular cartilage can be largely restated as the degradation of collagens and proteoglycans, which between them account for over 90% of the dry weight of cartilage. Approximately 95% of the collagen of articular cartilage is type II collagen, with types V, VI, IX, XI and, in calcified zones, type X collagen accounting for the remainder. By acting as linkers, several of the minor collagens may have an importance in maintaining the cartilagenous matrix that belies their low abundance. Cartilage proteoglycans are heterogeneous, but share a common basic structure in which glycosaminoglycan (GAG) chains are covalently bound to a core protein. The major type of proteoglycan present in articular cartilage has the ability to bind non-covalently to hyaluronic acid via a N-terminal binding domain. This interaction, which is stabilised by a link protein, results in the formation of very large aggregates vital to the biochemical and mechanical integrity of cartilage.

The extensive biochemical disruption of the cartilaginous matrix seen in advanced arthritis can occur as a result of surprisingly little enzymic attack. This is particularly true of the aggregating proteoglycans, because they are not covalently bound into the matrix. Instead they are sterically constrained by their large size within the collagenous meshwork of cartilage. As a result, loosening of this meshwork by limited collagenolysis, or removal of the hyaluronate binding domain by a single peptidolytic cleavage of the core protein, permits proteoglycans to diffuse from the cartilage. Hence, to understand the key mechanisms of cartilage destruction, it is not necessary to concern ourselves with the complete digestion of collagen and proteoglycan to small peptides and individual sugars. This review will thus concentrate on those proteinases which initiate the extracellular breakdown of cartilage, and largely ignore the subsequent steps through which their digestion products are more comprehensively degraded.

Pertinant to the present discussions is the observation that chondrocytes can reverse the depletion of proteoglycans from articular cartilage by synthesising replacement molecules. Replacement of collagen, on the contrary, may be imperfect. Thus the onset of substantial collagenolysis could signal the start of irreversible damage to the cartilage. In the present absence of reliable anti-erosive drugs, this culminates in the need for joint replacement surgery.

Despite the presence of large amounts of carbohydrate in the cartilaginous matrix, chondrolysis is initiated proteolytically. Much of the research effort in this area has been directed towards identifying proteinases capable of depolymerising cartilage collagens and proteoglycans, establishing their pathophysiological relevance, determining their cellular origin and delineating the mechanisms which regulate their activities. The structure of this review reflects these endeavours, with an emphasis of the author's main area of interest, the neutral metalloproteinases (NMPs).

Which proteinases degrade cartilage?: Type II collagen exists within cartilage as a highly cross-linked, insoluble polymer. It is susceptible to two forms of extracellular degradation (Murphy and Reynolds, 1985). The more direct process involves cleavage of the triple helical domain by specific collagenases. A more general mechanism involves a number of less specific proteinases. Although unable to degrade the triple helical structure of type II collagen, these enzymes remove the terminal, non-helical, telopeptides through which cross-linking occurs. Their actions tend both to solubilise individual collagen molecules and to facilitate their spontaneous denaturation into gelatin; denaturation is also favoured by the elevated temperature of an inflamed joint. Gelatin is a good substrate for a number of different proteinases. There also exist proteinases which degrade the minor collagens of articular cartilage (Gadher et al., 1988). As these enzymes remain to be clearly identified, they are not considered further in this paper.

Unlike the triple helical domain of type II collagen, the core proteins of cartilage proteoglycans are readily degraded by several different proteolytic enzymes. As the GAG chains sterically protect proteolytically susceptible sites on the core protein, digestion tends to occur at discrete locations with few GAG substituents. One such site of great significance occurs adjacent to the hyaluronate binding domain. When proteolysis occurs here, the proteoglycan molecules cannot aggregate in association with hyaluronic acid. As a result they are no longer restrained within the cartilage, despite losing only a tiny fraction of their mass.

Proteinases are classified according to the nature of their catalytic sites into the following four groups: aspartic, cysteine, serine and metallo. Members of the first two groups are usually lysosomal and have acidic pH optima. Members of the last two groups are usually extra-lysosomal and nearly always have pH optima close to neutral.

As shown in Table I, representatives from all four groups of proteinases have activity against type II collagen, proteoglycan or both, under in vitro conditions. Thus there is no lack of proteinases available for the digestion of the main macromolecules of the cartilaginous matrix. The problem is to determine which ones are pathophysiologically relevant in particular arthritides. This has proved a surprisingly difficult task. All the enzymes listed in Table I that have yet been measured, are present at higher concentrations at sites of cartilage resorption. This could indicate that they are all pathophysiologically important agents of cartilage breakdown. However, there are grounds for believing this not to be so. A good example is cathepsin D, which for a number of years was considered a major mediator of cartilage destruction in arthritis. In addition to degrading proteoglycans in vitro, it is present at elevated concentrations in the extracellular matrix of diseased cartilage (Sapolsky et al, 1973). However, despite earlier evidence to the contrary, Woessner (1973) demonstrated that cathepsin D had no activity against proteoglycan above pH 6. As the extracellular matrix of cartilage is buffered at a pH of around 7.4, cathepsin D would presumably be inactive in this environment. Although there are ways to argue around this limitation, further evidence against a role for cathepsin D in the extracellular resorption of cartilage came from inhibitor studies (Hembry et al, 1982). In view of these sorts of findings, cathepsin D has fallen out of fashion in the present context.

Nevertheless, other acidic enzymes, particularly cathepsins B and L are still actively discussed in this regard. Two types of argument are sometimes advanced to support the involvement of acidic proteinases in the digestion of an extracellular matrix that is ostensibly at a slightly alkaline pH. The first, a general claim applicable to all lysosomal hydrolases, is that the chondrocyte acidifies its immediate pericellular domain in a manner analogous to the ruffled border of the osteoclast. This hypothesis could help explain the pericellular nature of cartilage digestion that is often seen.

However, unless the release of lysosomal hydrolases were selective, we might expect to observe the pericellular digestion of GAGs through the secretion of lysosomal sulphatases and glycosidases into this domain. Such digestion has never been found, despite many attempts. Until the pH of the perichondrocytic domain has been measured, and the activities of acidic hydrolases present there have been assayed, this remains an untested hypothesis. A more specific claim, which applies at least to cathepsin B, is that certain acidic proteinases survive and retain some activity at neutral pH. Cathepsin B is present at elevated concentrations in human cartilage recovered from arthritic joints, and is considered, along with cathepsin L, a possible pathophysiological mediator of chondrolysis (Martel-Pelletier et al, 1990; Nguyen et al, 1990).

The probable involvement of serine and metalloproteinases in cartilage destruction is less controversial, albeit unproven. Both are active at the pH of the extracellular matrix and both are present at elevated concentrations in diseased cartilage. The best data apply to the NMPs, in particular collagenase, which are presently under intensive investigation as mediators of cartilage destruction. NMPs have been detected biochemically and immunologically at elevated concentrations in various joint tissues obtained both from human patients (e.g. Woolley et al, 1978; Martel-Pelletier et al, 1988) and from experimental animals (e.g. Ciosek and Harrity 1980; Pelletier et al, 1988). The latter studies have confirmed that NMP production is switched on early in the development of experimental arthritis, and that this is correlated with destruction of the extracellular matrix (Hasty et al, 1990). Under in vitro conditions in which chondrocytes degrade their surrounding cartilaginous matrix under the influence of interleukin-1 (IL-1), loss of proteoglycan from the matrix is reduced by non-toxic doses of certain chelators that inhibit NMPs (Arner et al, 1987; Smith et al, 1989). There are also preliminary in vivo data of this kind (Ishizue et al, 1984).

Furthermore, the sequences of protein fragments produced by the action of cartilage NMPs are consistent with degradation mediated by stromelysin (Nguyen et al, 1989).

TABLE I

PROTEINASES WHICH DEGRADE CARTILAGE MACROMOLECULES

				Substrate			
				Collagen*		Gelatin	Proteo-
Type	pH Optimum	Name	M.W. kDa	Direct	Indirect		glycan
Aspartic	Acidic	Cathepsin D	40	-	-	-	+
Cysteine	Acidic	Cathepsin B	25	-	+	+	+
		Cathepsin L	29	-	+	+	+
Serine	Neutral	Plasmin	90	-	-	+	+
		Elastase (Leucocyte)	28	-	+	+	+
		Cathepsin G	20	-	+	+	+
Metallo	Neutral	Collagenase (mesenchyme)	55	+	-	±	±
		Collagenase (neutrophil)	75	+	-	±	-
		Stromelysin	57	-	+	+	+
		Gelatinase (Type IV collagenase)	75	-	-	+	-
		Gelatinase (Type V collagenase)	97	-	-	+	-
		Elastase (macrophage)	22	-	-	-	+

*-The direct mode of type II collagen breakdown refers to cleavage across the triple helical domain of the molecule. The indirect mode refers to solubilisation through the removal of the terminal telopeptides whre cross-linking occurs. M.W.s of the three main types of NMPs refer to human proenzymes.

Recent data suggest that the list of NMPs given in Table I is incomplete. Molecular analysis has revealed the presence of a second stromelysin gene and a gene coding for a putative metalloproteinase which goes under the acronym "pump" (Muller et al, 1988). Others may await detection.

Most members of the NMP family share a 3-domain structure

comprising the propeptide domain, a catalytic domain containing a Zn atom and a C-terminal, disulphide bonded domain, which may help confer substrate specificity. The C-terminal domain contains about 200 amino acids and has homology to hemopexin and vitronectin. Pump lacks this domain and is a much smaller molecule. Comparison of the amino acid sequences of these NMPs has revealed considerable amino acid homology, including 3 conserved cysteine residues. Two of these occur in the C-terminal region, while the third is present in the pro-sequence that is lost upon activation. Both gelatinases have in their catalytic domain three repeats of a 58 amino acid, cysteine rich insertion with strong homology to the collagen binding domain of fibronectin. The larger gelatinase has an additional insertion of 53 amino acids at the C-terminus of this domain. This insertion shares homology with the α_2 chain of type V collagen.

Each of the NMPs is secreted as a latent proenzyme with the approximate M.W. shown in Table 1. Activation involves the proteolytic removal of a propeptide, as discussed in the next section. The activated enzymes cleave their substrates at the N-terminal side of hydrophobic residues.

It is possible that additional proteinases involved in the pathological resorption of cartilage remain to be identified. Azzo and Woessner (1986), for instance, have characterized an acid metalloproteinase from cartilage which degrades proteoglycans. T-lymphocytes also secrete a neutral, metalloproteoglycanase (Kammer et al, 1985). In addition calpains, which are calcium-dependent, neutral, cysteine proteinases normally involved in intracellular proteolysis, have been detected extracellularly in synovial fluid (Suzuki et al, 1990).

Although each enzyme discussed in this section has been considered separately, the physiological degradation of cartilage involves the combined activities of several proteinases acting together. There is clearly much scope for synergy and potentiation, particularly in the complex process of degrading the cross-linked, insoluble, polymeric type II collagen of the cartilagenous matrix.

<u>Cellular Sources of Chondrolytic Proteinases:</u> Proteinases present in normal and diseased joints are generated locally. In the absence of inflammation, the joint is populated by several types of mesenchymal cells. The synovium contains at least two types of cell, the 'type A' synoviocyte which resembles a macrophage and the 'type B' synoviocyte which is fibroblastic. Endothelial cells lining blood vessels within the synovium may constitute an additional source of intraarticular proteinases. Articular cartilage contains a sparse population of articular chondrocytes which, although considered to be of a single type, show morphological and biochemical variations depending upon their depth within the cartilage.

During inflammation, the joint becomes colonised by white blood cells migrating from blood vessels within the synovium. In acute episodes, large numbers of polymorphonuclear (PMN) leucocytes accumulate in the synovial fluid, where their concentration can be as high as 10^7 cells/ml. Few PMNs are found in the synovium. Here the predominant inflammatory cells are lymphocytes and macrophages, while the population of synovial fibroblasts is considerably augmented through cell division. Mast cells are also present, with hypervascularity of the synovium increasing the representation of endothelial cells. The repertoire of proteinases released from the most prominant of these types of cells in listed in Table II. Although mast cells release proteinases, mast cell extracts have not been found to digest collagen (Gruber et al, 1988) or proteoglycan (Johnson and Cawston, 1985). However, mast cell tryptase may activate latent collagenase (q.v.). Examination of Table II suggests that in the absence of inflammation, chondrolysis is predominantly mediated by NMPs, possibly in conjunction with the serine proteinase, plasmin, generated through the action of plasminogen activator.

Under acute inflammatory conditions, the presence of large numbers of PMN leucocytes introduces into the joint considerable amounts of serine proteinases. It has been estimated that PMNs can liberate as much as 8 mg per day of these enzymes into an acutely inflamed knee (Barrett, 1978). This calculation renders surprisingly the finding that cartilage destruction in antigen-induced arthritis is not reduced in PMN-depleted animals (Pettipher et al, 1988). During chronic inflammation, where the PMN concentration is low, NMPs are again likely to be the dominant proteinases of the extracellular matrix. It is important to realise that even without an inflammatory infiltrate, the resident mesenchymal cells of the joint have the capacity to secrete proteinases which degrade cartilage. Thus even in conditions like osteoarthritis, where inflammation is low or absent, excessive cartilage destruction may occur through the actions of locally synthesised proteolytic enzymes.

TABLE II

MAIN CELLULAR SOURCES OF PROTEINASES IN JOINTS

	Cell Type	Major Secreted Proteinases
Uninflamed Joints:	Chondrocyte Synoviocyte	Collagenase Gelatinase Stromelysin Plasminogen Activator
Inflamed Joints:	PMNs	Collagenase Gelatinase Elastase Cathepsin G Plasminogen Activator
	Macrophages	Collagenase Gelatinase Stromelysin Elastase Plasminogen Activator

Regulation of Extracellular Proteinase Activity: In general terms, the extracellular activities of the enzymes thus far discussed may be regulated at one or more of the four following stages: synthesis, secretion, activation and inhibition. Not all of them are subject to regulation at all of these levels.

Lysosomal hydrolases and the proteinases of PMN leucocytes are stored intracellularly. Their extracellular activities do not depend upon their rates of synthesis, but upon the rates at which they are released from the cell. The NMPs and plasminogen activator of mesenchymal cells and macrophages are quite different in this respect. Resting cells obtained from normal tissues spontaneously produce only low levels of these enzymes; indeed, their synthesis is sometimes undetectable. However, during the development of arthritis, synthesis is greatly augmented as a result of cellular activation. There is, however, no evidence that the rate of secretion of these enzymes is a regulatory parameter. Instead, NMPs are secreted as latent proenzymes lacking proteolytic activity. Their conversion to active proteinases constitutes an important, albeit imperfectly understood, point of control. All four classes of proteinase are further subject to regulation by extracellular inhibitors.

Synoviocytes and chondrocytes are activated by a number of soluble and particulate stimuli. Cultures of synovial fibroblasts increase their production of NMPs in response to interleukin-1 (IL-1), tumour necrosis factor (TNF), substance P, β-2 microglobulin, amyloid A and possibly epidermal growth factor. IL-1 also activates chondrocytes. TNF-α, while activating human articular chondrocytes, appears not to activate lapine articular chondrocytes. Fibroblast growth factor and platelet-derived growth factor do not induce NMPs in chondrocytes, but strongly potentiate the inductive effects of IL-1. Because of its potent activating properties, particular attention is presently being paid to IL-1. Although primarily a product of activated macrophages, IL-1 is contained within PMN leucocytes (Watanabe et al, 1989) and is also synthesised by synoviocytes (Wood et al, 1985) and chondrocytes (Ollivierre et al, 1986). Thus the intraarticular production of IL-1 need not depend upon the presence of inflammatory cells.

Particulate activators include the urate crystals of gouty joints (McMillan et al, 1981) and various other minerals, such as hydroxyapatite, present in other arthritides. Cellular activation by the cartilagenous wear debris found in osteoarthritis (Evans et al, 1981) illustrates one way in which the cartilagenous matrix, instead of just being a passive victim of chondrolysis, can fuel the disease process. Moreover, there is evidence that the soluble products of cartilage erosion also feed arthritogenic processes (Boniface et al, 1988). These findings raise the possibility that, under certain conditions, inflammation can be secondary to cartilage breakdown, contradicting the commonly held view that this only occurs the other way around. This mechanistic distinction between inflammation and cartilage breakdown has important therapeutic implications.

Cells can be de-activated as well as activated. Transforming growth factor-β, for instance, suppresses the synthesis of NMPs in chondrocytes (Chandrasekhar and Harvey, 1988). In addition, there exist inhibitors of synovial cell activation as well as specific antagonists of IL-1 and TNF-α (Arend and Dayer, 1990).

Induction of NMPs and plasminogen activators in synovial fibroblasts and chondrocytes is associated with increases in the abundances of their cognate mRNAs (Gross et al, 1984; Lin et al, 1988). There is increasing evidence that this reflects transcriptional control (Frisch and Ruley, 1987) although message stabilization may also occur (Brinckerhoff et al, 1986). Under in vitro conditions, the induction of collagenase, gelatinase and stromelysin is usually coordinate. However, recent data from ex vivo studies suggest that they are individually expressed in vivo.

Conversion of latent proenzymes to active NMPs occurs extracellularly. During this proteolytic process, the M.W. of the enzyme decreases by approximately 10 kDa as a propeptide of around 80 amino acids is cleaved from the N-terminus. Among the physiological activators of latent NMPs are plasmin and kallikrein which are themselves present in the serum as the latent precursors plasminogen and prokallikrein. Stromelysin activates procollagenase, while prostromelysin appears to have some ability to activate itself. Other activators of latent NMPs include cathepsin B and possibly mast cell tryptase (Gruber et al, 1988).

Joints contain a variety of proteinase inhibitors, some of which are systemic inhibitors derived from the circulation, while others are synthesized locally. The systemic inhibitor α_2-

macroglobulin is unusual in inhibiting proteinases of all four types. Although present at a concentration of around 2.5 mg/ml in plasma, its concentration in synovial fluid is limited by the large size of this 725,000 Da protein. However, the permeability of the synovial membrane increases during inflammation, permitting the inhibitor access to the joint. Nevertheless it remains sterically excluded from the matrix of intact cartilage. Other important systemic inhibitors of proteinases are α_1-proteinase inhibitor, a fairly general inhibitor of serine proteinases, and the more specific α_2-antiplasmin and α_1-antichymotrypsin, which also inhibits cathepsin G. Cysteine proteinases are inhibited by specific proteins occurring in both high and low molecular weight forms. Although present in serum, there is evidence of local synthesis within cartilage (Martel-Pelletier et al, 1990).

Because of the difficulty that the larger systemic inhibitors have in diffusing across the synovium and penetrating to the pericellular regions of cartilage, there has been increasing interest in proteinase inhibitors produced by chondrocytes. Best studied of these in the tissue inhibitor of metalloproteinases (TIMP) which inhibits collagenase, gelatinase and stromelysin (Cawston et al, 1981). Small amounts of TIMP occur in serum from which it was first purified and called β_1-anticollagenase. A glycoprotein of approximately 30 kDa, TIMP binds to NMPs with a K_d of around 10^{-10}M. A second TIMP molecule has recently been identified (Stetler-Stevenson et al, 1989), which possesses around 40-50% amino acid homology to TIMP-1. TIMP-2 is an unglycosylated protein with a M.W. of approximately 20 kDa. SDS-substrate gel analysis has also detected three other inhibitors of metalloproteinases, known as IMP-1 (M.W. 22,000), IMP-2 (M.W. 19,000) and IMP-3 (M.W. 16,500) (Apodaca et al, 1990). It is not yet known whether articular chondrocytes synthesize TIMP-2 or the IMPs.

<u>Other Roles for Proteinases in Chondrolysis</u>: Thus far, we have been discussing proteinases in terms of their ability to degrade collagen and proteoglycan. However, they may also aid the breakdown of cartilage indirectly, one instance being the

proteolytic activation of latent proenzymes as mentioned in the last section. There are several other examples which are listed in Table III. Particularly interesting is the recent report that collagenase, cathepsin G and elastase convert the inactive, 31-kDa precursor of IL-1β to the 17 kDa active form (Hazuda et al, 1990).

TABLE III

ACCESSORY ROLES FOR PROTEINASES IN CHONDROLYSIS

Activation of latent proenzymes
Destruction or saturation of inhibitors
Generation of antigenic products
Activation of synovial fibroblasts
Activation of complement
Conversion of pro-interleukin-1

Points of potential therapeutic intervention: Although the pharmacologic effort in arthritis therapy has traditionally addressed the problem of inflammation, there are grounds for suggesting a re-targeting of resources towards specifically protecting the articular cartilage. Destruction of cartilage is the major pathological lesion in many forms of arthritis, and the one leading to irreversible loss of joint function. As I have tried to emphasize in this review, cartilage breakdown and inflammation can occur independently of each other. Furthermore, inflammation may, in certain circumstances, be secondary to cartilage destruction. Thus pharmacologically inhibiting articular inflammation need not necessarily block cartilage destruction. Under these circumstances, therapeutically modulating the activities of the proteinases discussed in this paper is a better approach to protecting the articular cartilage. From the foregoing discussion it appears that this may be achieved in several ways.

Firstly, the activators which induce the cellular synthesis of NMPs could be eliminated or neutralised. Progress in this direction is indicated by the recent characterisation of antagonists of IL-1 and TNF-α (Arend and Dayer, 1990). Secondly, the responses of cells to these activators could be subdued.

TGF-β, for example, interacts with chondrocytes to suppress their induction of NMPs in response to IL-1. Dexamethasone and other steroids also inhibit NMP production. Thirdly, enzyme inhibitors might be employed to reduce the extracellular activities of proteinases within cartilage. This could be achieved by stimulating the endogenous synthesis of native inhibitors, or by administering natural or synthetic inhibitors. Recent progress in the molecular characterisation of the naturally occurring inhibitors will aid the design of drugs suitable for pharmacologic use (Henderson et al, 1990). In view of the metabolic isolation of articular cartilage, their successful application will require improved drug delivery systems.

Acknowledgements: I am grateful to Miss J. Galea-Lauri and Dr. Geethãni Bandara for critically reading earlier drafts of this paper. I also thank Mrs. Lou Duerring and Miss Heather Watson for their considerable efforts in preparing this paper.

This article was written while the author was in receipt of a Senior International Fellowship (No. 1F06 TW01607) from the Fogarty International Center of the National Institutes of Health.

References:

(Page restrictions limit the number of references cited).

REFERENCES

Apodaca, G., Rutka, J.T., Bouhana, K., Berens, M.E., Giblin, J. R., Rosenblum, M.L., McKerrow, J.H. and Banda, M.J. (1990) Expression of metalloproteinases and metalloproteinase inhibitors by fetal astrocytes and glioma cells. Cancer Res. 50 2322-2329.

Arend, W.P. and Dayer, J.M. (1990) Cytokines and cytokine inhibitors or antagonists in rheumatoid arthrisit. Arthritis Rheum. 33 305-315.

Arner, E.C., Darnell, L.R., Pratta, M.A., Newton, R.C., Ackerman, N.R. and Galbraith, W. (1987) Effect of antiinflammatory drugs on human interleukin-1-induced cartilage degradation. Agents Actions 21 334-336.

Azzo, W. and Woessner, J.F. (1986) Purification and characterization of an acid metalloproteinase from human articular cartilage. J. Biol. Chem. 261 5434-5441.

Barrett, A.J. (1978) The possible role of neutrophil proteinases in damage to articular cartilage. Agents Actions 8 11-17.

Boniface, R.J., Cain, P.R. and Evans, C.H. (1988) Articular responses to purified cartilage proteoglycans. Arthritis Rheum. 31 258-266.

Brinckerhoff, C.E., Plucinska, I.M., Sheldon, L.A. and O'Connor, G.T. (1986) Half-life of synovial cell collagenase mRNA is modulated by phorbol myristate acetate but not by all-transretinoic acid or dexamethasone. Biochemistry 25 6378-6384.

Cawston, T.E., Galloway, W.A., Mercer, E., Murphy, G. and Reynolds, J.J. (1981) Purification of rabbit bone inhibitor of collagenase. Biochem. J. 195 159-165.

Chandrasekhar, S. and Harvey, A.K. (1988) Transforming growth factor-β is a potent inhibitor of IL-1 induced protease activity and cartilage proteoglycan degradation. Biochem. Biophys. Res. Commun. 157 1352-1359.

Ciosek, C.P. and Harrity, T.W. (1980) Cartilage-associated collagenolytic activity in rabbits with antigen-induced chronic synovitis. J. Lab. Clin. Med. 96 460-469.

Evans, C.H., Mears, D.C. and Cosgrove, J.L. (1981) Release of neutral proteinases from mononuclear phagocytes and synovial cells in response to cartilaginous wear particles in vitro. Biochim. Biophys. Acta 677 287-294.

Frisch, S.M. and Ruley, H.E. (1987) Transcription from the stromelysin promoter is induced by interleukin-1 and repressed by dexamethasone. J. Biol. Chem. 262 16300-16304.

Gadher, S.J., Eyre, D.R., Duance, V.C., Wotton, S.F., Heck, L.W., Schmid, T.M. and Wolley, D.E. (1988) Susceptibility of cartilage collagens type II, IX, X and XI to human synovial collagenase and neutrophil elastase. Eur. J. Biochem. 175 1-7.

Gross, R.H., Sheldon, L.S., Fletcher, C.F. and Brinckerhoff, C.E. (1984) Isolation of a collagenase cDNA clone and measurement of changing collagenase mRNA levels during induction in rabbit synovial fibroblasts. Proc. Natl. Acad. Sci. USA 81 1981-1985.

Gruber, B.L., Schwartz, Z.B., Ramanerthy, N.S., Irani, A.M. and Marchese, M.J. (1988) Activation of latent rheumatoid synovial collagenase by human mast cell tryptase. J. Immunol. 140 3936-3942.

Hasty, K.A., Reife, R.A., Kang, A.H. and Stuart, J.M. (1990) The role of stromelysin in the cartilage destruction that accompanies inflammatory arthritis. Arthritis Rheum. 33 388-397.

Hazuda, D.J., Strickler, J., Kueppers, F., Simon, P.L. and Young, P.R. (1990) Processing of precursor interleukin-1β and inflammatory disease. J. Biol. Chem. 265 6318-6322.

Hembry, R.M., Knight, C.G., Dingle, J.J. and Barrett, A.J. (1982) Evidence that cathepsin D is not responsible for the resorption of cartilage matrix in culture. Biochim. Biophys. Acta 714 307-312.

Henderson, B., Docherty, A.J.P. and Beeley, N.R.A. (1990) Design of inhibitors of articular cartilage destruction. Drugs of the future 15 495-506.

Ishizue, K.K., Ehrlich, M.G. and Mankin, H.J. (1984) Drug induced inhibition of proteoglycanase activity in the Hulth-Telhag model. Trans. Orthop. Res. Soc. 9 343.

Johnson, D.A. and Cawston, T.A. (1985) Human lung mast cell tryptase fails to activate procollagenase or degrade proteoglycan. Biochem. Biophys. Res. Commun. 132 453.

Kammer, G.M., Sapolsky, A.I. and Malemud, C.J. (1985) Secretion of an articular cartilage proteoglycan-degrading enzyme activity by murine T-lymphocytes in vitro. J. Clin. Invest. 76 395-402.

Lin, C.W., Phillips, S.L., Brinckerhoff, C.E., Georgescu, H.I., Bandara, G. and Evans, C.H. (1988) Induction of collagenase mRNA in lapine articular chondrocytes by synovial factors and interleukin-1. Arch. Biochem. Biophys. 264 351-354.

Martel-Pelletier, J., Cloutier, J.M. and Pelletier, J.P. (1990) Cathepsin B and cysteine protease inhibitors in human osteoarthritis. J. Orthop. Res. 8 336-344.

Martel-Pelletier, J., Pelletier, J.P. and Malemud, C.J. (1988) Activation of neutral metalloprotease in human osteoarthritic knee cartilage: evidence for degradation in the core protein of sulphated proteoglycan. Ann. Rheum. Dis. 47 801-808.

McMillan, R.M., Vater, C.A., Hasselbacher, P., Hahn, J. and Harris, E.D. (1981) Induction of collagenase and prostaglandin synthesis in synovial fibroblasts treated with monosodium urate crystals. J. Pharm. Pharmacol. 33 382-383.

Muller, D., Quantin, B., Gesnel, M.C., Millon-Collard, R., Abecassis, J. and Breathnach, R. (1988) The collagenase gene family in humans consists of at least four members. Biochem. J. 253 187-192.

Murphy, G. and Reynolds, J.J. (1985) Current views of collagen degradation. BioEssays 2 55-60.

Nguyen, Q., Mort, J.S. and Roughley, P.J. (1990) Cartilage proteoglycan aggregate is degraded more extensively by cathepsin L than by cathepsin B. Biochem. J. 266 569-573.

Nguyen, Q., Murphy, G., Roughley, P.J. and Mort, J.S. (1989) Degradation of proteoglycan aggregate by a cartilage metalloproteinase. Biochem. J. 259 61-67.

Ollivierre, F., Gubler, U., Towle, C., Laurencin, C. and Treadwell, B.V. (1986) Expression of IL-1 genes in human and bovine chondrocytes: a mechanism for autocrine control of cartilage matrix degradation. Biochem. Biophys. Res. Commun. 141 904-911.

Pelletier, J.P., Martel-Pelletier, J., Altman, R.D., Ghandur-Mnaymneh, L., Howell, D.S. and Woessner, J.F. (1983) Collagenolytic activity and collagen matrix breakdown of the articular cartilage in the Pond-Nuki dog model of osteoarthritis. Arthritis Rheum. 26 866-874.

Pettipher, E.R., Henderson, B., Moncada, S. and Higgs, G.A. (1988) Leucocyte infiltration and cartilage proteoglycan loss in immune arthritis in the rabbit. Br. J. Pharmacol. 95 169-176.

Sapolsky, A.I., Altman, R.D., Woessner, J.F. and Howell, D.S. (1973) The action of cathepsin D in human articular cartilage on proteoglycans. J. Clin. Invest. 52 624-633.

Smith, R.J., Rohloff, N.A., Sam, L.M., Justen, J.M., Deibel, M.R. and Cornette, J.C. (1989) Recombinant human interleukin-1α and recombinant human interleukin-1β stimulate cartilage matrix degradation and inhibit glycosaminoglycan synthesis. Inflammation 13 367-381.

Stetler-Stevenson, W.G., Krutzch, H.C. and Liotta, L.A. (1989) Tissue inhibitor of metalloproteinase (TIMP-2). A new member of the metalloproteinase inhibitor family. J. Biol. Chem. 264 17374-17378.

Susuki, K., Shimizu, K., Hamamoto, T., Nakagawa, Y., Hamakubo, T. and Yamamuro, T. (1990) Biochemical demonstration of calpins and calpastatin in osteoarthritic synovial fluid. Arthritis Rheum. 33 728-732.

Watanabe, S., Georgescu, H.I., Kuhns, D.B. and Evans, C.H. (1989) Chondrocyte activation by a putative interleukin-1 derived from lapine polymorphonuclear leukocytes. Arch. Biochem. Biophys. 270 69-76.

Woessner, J.F. (1973) Purification of cathepsin D from cartilage and uterus, and its action on the proteinpolysaccharide complex of cartilage. J. Biol. Chem. 248 1634-1641.

Wood, D.D., Ihrie, E.J. and Hammerman, D. (1985) Release of interleukin-1 from human synovial tissue in vitro. Arthritis Rheum. 28 853-862.

Woolley, D.E., Harris, E.D., Mainardi, C.L. and Brinckerhoff, C.E. (1978) Collagenase immunolocalization in cultures of rheumatoid synovial cells. Science 200 773-775.

AAS 32
Drugs in Inflammation

RECOGNITION OF IL1-ACTIVATED CHONDROCYTES IN PORCINE ARTICULAR CARTILAGE

M. Elisabeth Davies[1], Alan Horner[1] and Burkart Franz[2]

[1] Strangeways Research Laboratory, Worts' Causeway, Cambridge, CB1 4RN, U.K.

[2] Institut für Mikrobiologie and Tierseuchen der Tierärztliche Hochschule, Hannover, B.R.D.

SUMMARY: A polyclonal antiserum has been raised against interleukin 1 (IL1)-induced epitopes on the surface of porcine articular chondrocytes. Using this antiserum in immunolocalization studies we have been able to identify individual chondrocytes *in situ* both in experimentally activated articular cartilage and in pathological tissue from pigs with induced polyarthritis.

INTRODUCTION

The mechanisms involved in the control of connective tissue turnover, with particular reference to the mediators of the articular damage characteristic of rheumatoid and osteoarthritis are not fully understood. Although it is generally accepted that the catabolic cytokines IL1α, IL1β and tumour necrosis factor (TNFα) play a major role in chondrocyte-induced cartilage matrix resorption, the second messengers involved have not yet been fully elucidated. We assume that cell surface receptor binding of such cytokines "activates the chondrocytes leading indirectly to localized degradation of their surrounding matrix. As a means of identifying individual cytokine "activated" chondrocytes we have raised an antiserum against IL1-induced surface epitopes which we have shown to be a marker of IL1 activation (Dingle, Davies, Mativi and Middleton, 1990).

In this study we have used the antiserum to investigate the response of chondrocytes to IL1 under both experimental and pathological conditions.

MATERIALS AND METHODS

Antiserum: A polyclonal antiserum was raised in rabbits against IL1α-treated porcine articular chondrocytes and rendered specific for IL1-induced surface epitopes by exhaustive adsorption with normal untreated chondrocytes as previously described (Dingle et al., 1990).

Culture conditions: Chondrocytes were released from porcine articular cartilage by enzymic digestion, grown up to confluence and IL1 treated as previously described (Dingle et al., 1990). Explants of adult porcine articular cartilage were co-cultured with human rheumatoid or porcine synovium essentially as described by Fell and Jubb (1977).

The porcine model for rheumatoid arthritis: Five pigs were infected intraperitoneally with 5×10^6 colony-forming units of *Erysipelothrix rhusiopathiae* strain T28. This strain has been isolated from swine suffering from chronic Erysipelas infection and was found to be highly virulent for mice, rats and pigs (Bisping et al., 1968, Schulz et al., 1975) Infected pigs showed clinical signs of Erysipelas infection (body temperature > 41.5°C, apathy, stiffness, reluctance to move, and mild to moderate swelling of knee joints). At post mortem examination 8 weeks post-infection arthritic lesions or inflammation of cardiac valves were detected in all animals.

Immunohistological methods

(i) Immunofluorescent localization: Chondrocyte monolayers or frozen of porcine catilage (4-6μm thick) were incubated with primary antibody (rabbit anti-IL1 activated porcine chondrocyte serum or rabbit anti-human recombinant IL1α or IL1ß, dil 1:200), secondary antibody (FITC-conjugated pig anti-rabbit Ig serum (Dako), dil 1:200), counter-stained and viewed as previously described (Dingle et al., 1990).

(ii) Electron microscopy: Ultrastructural localization was kindly performed by Dr Audrey M. Glauert at Strangeways Research Laboratory using standard techniques (Glauert, Oliver and Thorne, 1980).

RESULTS

Activation of porcine chondrocytes in monolayer culture by IL1: Monolayer cultures of porcine chondrocytes showed uniform surface fluorescence after treatment with 2ng/ml IL1-α for 4-16 hr. Untreated monolayers were negative. The number of positive chondrocytes was found to be variable, and at no time were all cells stained.

Electron microscopical examination of the chondrocytes confirmed binding of antibody to the plasma membrane (Fig. 1).

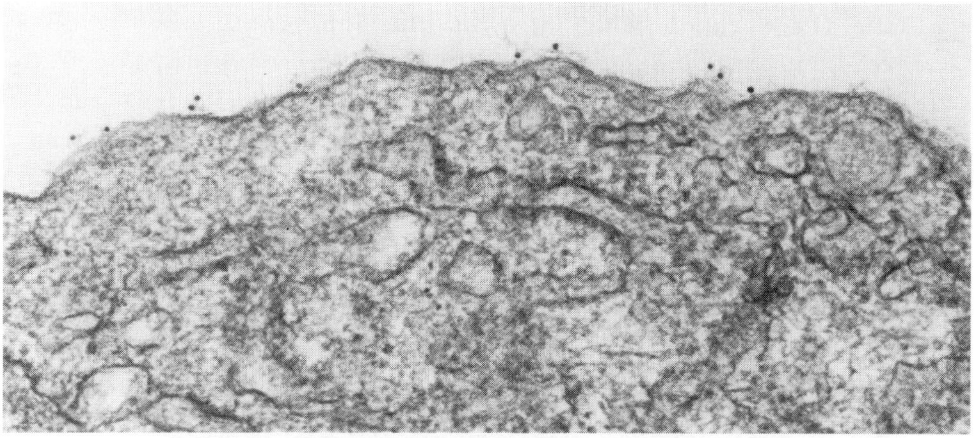

Fig.1. Electron-micrograph of 4hr IL1-α treated chondrocyte monolayer culture demonstrating pre-embeddding immunoreactivity with antiserum raised against IL1-induced surface epitopes, and 10nm gold-labelled goat anti-rabbit Ig serum (BioCell).

Activation of porcine chondrocytes by synovial tissue: Frozen sections of the co-cultures were examined for fluorescent staining after incubation with the antiserum raised against IL1-activated porcine chondrocytes. We observed that when porcine articular cartilage was co-cultured with porcine synovium for 4 days the chondrocytes at the articular surface immediately adjacent to the synovium were activated, exhibiting intense surface staining. Chondrocytes distant from the synovium, in the mid and hypertrophic zones were negative, being visualized by their counter-stained nuclei. Three samples of human rheumatoid synovium appeared to be more stimulatory than porcine synovium as indicated by activation of chondrocytes well into the mid zone. There was no evidence of intracellular staining.

The presence of both IL1-α and IL1-ß in the human rheumatoid synovial tissue was confirmed by immunolocalization using specific antisera (Cistron, Lab Impex).

Activation of chondrocytes in the porcine arthritis model: Using normal histological staining techniques we demonstrated that articular cartilage removed from an affected joint exhibited the morphological changes characteristic of rheumatoid arthritis i.e. infiltration by "fingers" of inflammatory synovial tissue, pannus formation and localized depletion of matrix proteoglycan. In the same tissue we found that the majority of chondrocytes throughout the articular and mid-zone regions were expressing IL1-induced surface epitopes, as recognised by the antiserum raised against IL1-α treated porcine chondrocytes (Fig.2). Tissue from healthy pigs showed no immunostaining with the antiserum.

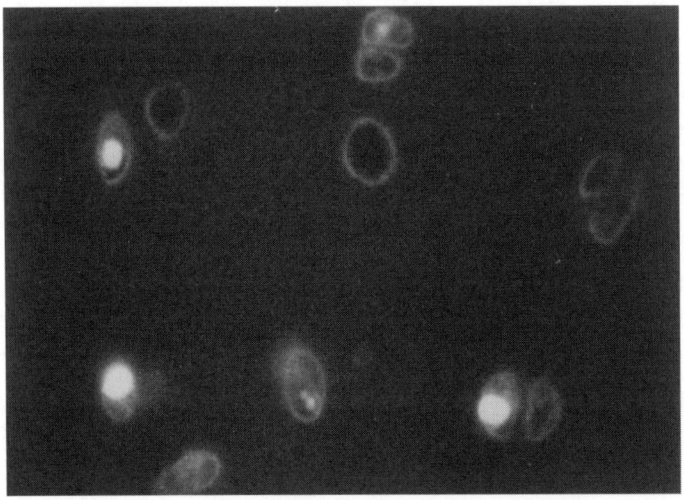

Fig.2. Immunolocalization of IL1-activated chondrocytes in articular cartilage from an affected joint of a pig suffering from *Erysipelothrix rhusiopathiae*-induced polyarthritis.

DISCUSSION

In this study we have used an antiserum raised against IL1-induced surface epitopes to observe the response of individual chondrocytes to cytokine activation. This novel method has demonstrated the experimental activation of chondrocytes *in situ* in cartilage by synovial tissue shown to be producing IL1, and has confirmed the usefulness of the antiserum as a marker of IL1 activation.

We have also shown that this approach can be applied to *in vivo* studies on pathological tissues. Our preliminary observations on the pig Erysipelas model (which is considered to be one of the best animal models for human R.A.) indicate that we will be able to use the antiserum to investigate the early events of cytokine activation *in vivo*, with particular reference to the interactions between synovium and cartilage.

REFERENCES

Bisping, W., Böhm, K.H., and Weiland, E. (1968). Zur derzeitigen Verlaufsform des chronischen Rotlaufs beim Schwein. Teil III: Bakteriologische und serologische Ergebnisse. Dtsch. Tierärztl. Wochenschr. 75, 445-50.

Dingle, J.T., Davies, M.E., Mativi, B.Y., and Middleton, H.F. (1990). Immunohistological identification of interleukin-1 activated chondrocytes. Ann. Rheum. Dis. (in the Press).

Fell, H.B., and Jubb, R.W. (1977). The effect of synovial tissue on the breakdown of articular cartilage in organ culture. Arth. Rheum. 20, 1359-71.

Glauert, A.M., Oliver, R.C., amd Thorne, K.J.I. (1980). The interaction of human eosinophils and neutrophils with non-phagocytosable surfaces: a model for studying cell mediated immunity in schistosomiasis. Parasitology 80, 525-37.

Schulz, L.C., Drommer, W., Seidler, D., Erhard, H., Leimbeck, R., and Weiss, R. (1975). Experimenteller Rotlauf bei verschiedenen Spezies als Modell einer systemischen Bindegewebskrankheit. II. Chronische Phase unter besonderer Berücksichtigung der Polyarthritis. Beitr. Pathol. 154, 27-51.

AAS 32
Drugs in Inflammation

IN VIVO EVIDENCE FOR A KEY ROLE OF Il-1 IN CARTILAGE DESTRUCTION IN EXPERIMENTAL ARTHRITIS

Wim B van den Berg, Fons AJ van de Loo, Ivan Otterness*, Onno Arntz and Leo AB Joosten.

Dept of Rheumatology, University Hospital Nijmegen, 6525 GA Nijmegen, The Netherlands, * Immunology Division, Pfizer Central Research, Groton CT, USA.

SUMMARY

Cartilage destruction in murine antigen induced arthritis is characterized by enhanced degradation of proteoglycans and inhibition of chondrocyte proteoglycan synthesis. Within this model common NSAIDs only suppress joint swelling, and to some extent granulocyte infiltration, but leave the process of cartilage destruction undisturbed. Evidence is now accumulating that the vast amount of activated granulocytes in the joint space are of minor importance, and that interleukin-1 (IL-1) is the key mediator in this process. Treatment of mice with neutralizing antibodies against IL-1 resulted in relief of chondrocyte proteoglycan synthesis inhibition and prevented matrix destruction. This indicates that it makes sense to focus future therapy on elimination of IL-1.

Antigen induced arthritis (AIA) is a unilateral, allergic type of joint inflammation, which is accompanied by marked cartilage destruction (1). The arthritis is induced by intraarticular injection of an antigen in the knee joint of a preimmunized animal, and the chronic synovitis is determined by the degree of antigen retention in the knee joint and the presence of adequate cell mediated immunity against the retained antigen (2). The model bears resemblance with rheumatoid arthritis in terms of the immune infiltrate in the synovium, immune complex deposits in the superficial cartilage layers, and poor responsiveness to NSAIDs (3,4). The latter drugs only suppress joint swelling, but do not protect against joint destruction in AIA. In marked contrast, the joint destruction in other arthritis models like adjuvant arthritis or collagen induced arthritis appears rather sensitive to NSAIDs, making findings with new drugs in these models however of poor predictive value for rheumatoid arthritis.

Evidence is now accumulating that IL-1 may play an important role in the process of cartilage destruction in allergic joint inflammation. The potency of IL-1 to cause cartilage destruction in vitro is beyond doubt, and recent studies also provided evidence that IL-1 could cause marked cartilage destruction in vivo (5,6). In fact, the histopathology of the synovium and the metabolic changes in the articular cartilage after repeated IL-1 injections remarkably resembled the changes noted in AIA.
It remained however to be seen whether IL-1 is the dominant mediator in a real arthritic process. We therefor started studies in the model of antigen induced arthritis aimed at elimination or blocking of IL-1 and subsequent analysis of the impact on the articular cartilage damage.
One approach would be to administer drugs which selectively inhibit IL-1 production or action. In addition, antibodies are now available against the IL-1 receptor, and even more promising, an IL-1 receptor antagonist (IL-1ra) has recently been cloned. Although straight forward, the latter approaches of receptor blockade are hampered by the fact that the antibodies do not easily penetrate cartilage, and that high receptor occupancy is needed to block IL-1 signaling. It is generally agreed that IL-1 already exerts an optimal effect at a receptor occupancy below 5%.
A third approach is to interfere with IL-1 action by repeated administration of neutralizing anti-IL-1 antibodies. Antibodies against murine recombinant IL-1a,b (mrIL-1a,b) were raised in goats and rabbits by Ivan Otterness. Neutralizing potency was proven in an in vitro IL-1 assay (NOB-1 cell

line). Moreover, a single injection of 200 ul antiserum completely prevented the systemic effects of a subsequent injection of a dose up to 1 ng mrIL-1 in mice.

Antigen induced arthritis was elicited by intraarticular injection of 60 ug mBSA in the knee joint and the animals were treated with antiserum at days -2, 0 and 2. Two control groups were used: a non-treated group and a group receiving a similar amount of normal serum. Joint inflammation was followed by [99m]-Technetium uptake measurements of the knee joints at days 2 and 4, and chondrocyte proteoglycan synthesis was measured ex vivo by [35S]-sulfate incorporation in isolated patellae.

Joint inflammation was significantly decreased in both serum treated groups, with slightly lower values found in the anti-IL-1 treated group compared to the control serum group (Table 1). It indicates that serum treatment in this heavy regimen is anti-inflammatory per se and this finding may relate to the observations in rheumatoid arthritis showing beneficial effects of mere immunoglobulin treatment.

The most important observation in this experiment was however the impact of anti-IL-1 treatment on the articular cartilage. Still marked inhibition of chondrocyte proteoglycan synthesis in the proper control group, and almost complete relief of this inhibition in the anti-IL-1 treated group (fig 1). Histology on total joint sections further confirmed the protective effect of anti-IL-1 treatment on cartilage proteoglycan loss, which normally is a combination of enhanced degradation and marked inhibition of synthesis of new proteoglycan. For comparison, the lack of relief of synthesis inhibiton in PMN-depleted mice is included in figure 1. The latter observation further underlines that mere suppression of joint inflammation, as observed in the control serum treated group and in the PMN-depleted mice, does not necessarily yield protection against cartilage damage. It indicates that although certain aspects of the inflammatory process are suppressed, the damaging process, probably IL-1 mediated, may

Table 1. Effect of anti-IL-1 treatment on joint swelling in AIA.

Treatment	Tc uptake (R/L)	
	day 2	day 4
-	2.51 ± 0.23	1.52 ± 0.15
Control goat	1.94 ± 0.47	1.28 ± 0.30
Goat anti-IL-1	1.72 ± 0.32	1.14 ± 0.10

200 ul serum was given subc at days -2, 0 and 2 Values represent joint inflammation in the right arthritic joint (± SD)

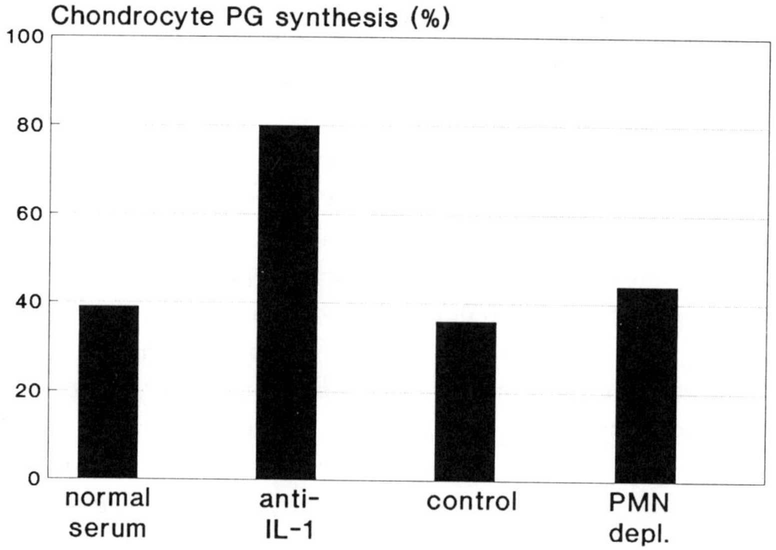

Fig 1. Chondrocyte proteoglycan synthesis was measured in in the arthritic patellar cartilage, isolated at day 4 and expressed as % of the synthesis in the normal contralateral joint. An additional group was treated at day -4 with 750 rad total body irradiation to deplete PMNs (>95%). PMN influx was abolished, but inhibition of synthesis remained.

proceed undisturbed. The latter situation seems also apparent in a number of rheumatoid arthritis patients, where drug treatment sometimes provides pain relief and reduction of joint swelling, suggestive for proper control of the inflammatory process, but X ray analysis in a later stage unfortunately shows progression of joint destruction.

Our data provide substantial evidence that it makes sense to focus future treatment on IL-1 elimination, or at least to combine treatments aimed to controll both the inflammatory signs and the destructive process. From a scientific point of view it is worthwhile to further discriminate between the potential role of either IL-1a or IL-1b. It is not to be expected that proper development of a synthetic IL-1 receptor antagonist would benefit from this, since the affinity of both forms of the IL-1 for the IL-1 receptor appears to be similar. It remains to be seen whether drugs can be developed which selectively inhibit the production/release/activation of IL-1a or IL-1b. Furthermore, it seems appropriate to investigate whether the production of endogenous IL-1ra can be modulated.

REFERENCES

1. Kruijsen MWM, van den Berg WB, van de Putte LBA. Significance of severity and duration of murine antigen induced arthritis for cartilage proteoglycan synthesis and chondrocyte death. Arthritis Rheum 26: 813, 1985
2. van den Berg WB, van de Putte LBA, Zwarts WA, Joosten LAB. Electrical charge of the antigen determines intraarticular antigen handling and chronicity of arthritis in mice. J Clin Invest 74: 1850, 1984
3. de Vries BJ, van den Berg WB. Impact of NSAIDs on murine antigen induced arthritis I: an investigation of antiinflammatory and chondroprotective effects. J Rheumatol 16: 10, 1989
4. Hunneyball IM, Crossley MJ, Spowage M. Pharmacological studies on antigen induced arthritis in BALB/c mice. Agents and Actions 18: 384, 1986
5. van de Loo AAJ, van den Berg WB. Effects of recombinant IL -1 on synovial joint in mice: measurement of patellar cartilage metabolism and joint inflammation. Ann Rheum Dis 49: 238, 1990
6. van Beuningen HM, Arntz OJ, van den Berg WB. In vivo effects of IL-1 on articular cartilage: disturbance of proteoglycan metabolism is more prolonged in old mice. Arthritis Rheum, in press.

AAS 32
Drugs in Inflammation

AN ANTI-CD4 ANTIBODY FOR TREATMENT OF CHRONIC INFLAMMATORY ARTHRITIS

F. Emmrich[1], G. Horneff[2], W. Becker[3], W. Lüke[4], A. Potocnik[1], U. Kanzy[5], J.R. Kalden[2] and G. Burmester[2]

Max-Planck-Society, Clinical Research Unit for Rheumatology[1] at the Institute for Clinical Immunology and Rheumatology[2], Dept. of Medicine III and Dept. of Nuclear Medicine[3] at the University of Erlangen-Nürnberg, German Primate Center Göttingen[4], Behringwerke, Marburg, FRG[5]

SUMMARY: Monoclonal antibodies (mAb) to the CD4 surface molecule inhibit the function of CD4^{+} T cells in vitro and have been used for treatment of autoimmune diseases in several animal models. Recently, an anti-CD4 mAb has been described that improved the clinical situation of rheumatoid arthritis (RA) patients although no change in laboratory parameters could be observed (6). Here, we report on a different high-affinity anti-CD4 mAb (MAX.16H5) and its use for treatment of RA. Reduction of the Ritchie index, morning stiffness and the number of swollen joints demonstrated the clinical benefits of the therapy. In addition, laboratory parameters like ESR, CRP, and rheumatoid factor were reduced in 6/12 treatments. A rapid depletion of CD4^{+} T cells was observed in all patients which reached a minimum 1 hour after administration. However, efficacy of treatment did not correlate with T cell depletion. The antibody accumulates at the site of inflamed joints as detected by 99m-Tc-labelling. Affected digital joints were detected earlier by virtue of helper T cell imaging than by conventional bone scans.

INTRODUCTION

Soluble anti-CD4 antibodies can inhibit T cell activation quite efficiently and have been used in several animal models for the suppression of T-cell-mediated autoimmune diseases (4). Furthermore, induction of peripheral T cell tolerance has been demonstrated in vivo by injecting the antigen during an anti-CD4 treatment interval (5). Therefore, anti-CD4 treatment appears to be a novel and promising therapeutical approach. It leaves CD8^{+}-T cells unaffected, thus protecting the defense against many infectious diseases which might interfere with a conventional immunosuppressive therapy. On the other hand, $CD4^+$-T cells are the most critical elements for the induction and maintenance of many experimental autoimmune diseases and some evidence exists for a similar role with human autoimmune diseases, although in most cases the causative agent is not known. Clinical improvement of RA has been demonstrated recently by anti-CD4 treatment (6), although significant changes of laboratory parameters could not be observed. Here we demonstrate the use of a new anti-CD4 mAb in RA treatment.

MATERIAL AND METHODS

10 patients suffering from severe and active rheumatoid arthritis were selected according the the ACR criteria (1). All patients had proved resistant to conventional therapy (Methotexate, D-penicillamine, Gold). Treatment was performed with the anti-CD4 mAb MAX.16H5 (IgG1). This reagent was produced, purified and tested following the guide lines of the German "Gesellschaft für Immunologie" (2). Flow cytometry was performed with an EPICS 753 (Coulter, Co. Hialeah, Fl. USA) using mAbs as indicated in the legend of Fig. 1. For imaging the mAb was prepared according to the Schwarz method (3) and Tc-99m-pertechnetate was added immediately before application.

RESULTS AND DISCUSSION

MAX.16H5 was selected for therapeutical use because of its high affinity to CD4 (K_D=5x10^{-10}M) as described previously (7). It modulates CD4 very efficiently as compared to other established anti-CD4 mAbs although not totally. In Fig.1 partial reduction of the mean fluorescence intensity is demonstrated with MAX.16H5. For comparison an anti-CD3 mAb is shown that totally modulates the corresponding T cell surface molecule.

MAX.16H5 was injected in a dosage of 0.3 mg/kg/day for seven days (8). It efficiently depleted circulating $CD4^+$ T cells to less than 100 cells/μl one hour after administration. In two thirds of the cases, the clinical situation of the patients could be improved as judged by the reduction of the Ritchie index, and by a reduced number of swollen joints with a duration of the clinical benefits lasting for 4 to 8 weeks. Indicators of inflammation including ESR (erythrocyte sedimentation rate) and CRP (c-reactive protein) were significantly decreased after 6/12 treatments as was the rheumatoid factor level (RF) in those patients. This change in laboratory parameters induced by MAX.16H5 seems to be unique for this antibody and has not been described with other anti-CD4 therapy trials (8). However, $CD4^+$ T cell depletion did not correlate with the efficacy of therapy as shown in Table 1. It has been demonstrated that anti-CD4 mAbs could reduce primary antibody responses at doses that did not cause depletion (9) or when the antibody was administered as an $F(ab)_2$ fragment (10). These data might indicate that functional blockade of the CD4 antigen as causative mechanism rather than inhibition by reduction of helper cells. It would be compatible with the view that helper cell depletion is not an absolute requirement for an effective anti-CD4 treatment.

No adverse effects were seen except in two cases showing chills and moderate rises in body temperature at the initial treatment. In two cases, patients were treated a second time after 3 months with more pronounced improvement of the disease. Since human anti-mouse antibodies remained at a low titer repeated treatments appear possible (11). Conventional second line anti-rheumatic therapy becomes effective only after 1-2 months of treatment whereas anti-CD4 induced an immediate beneficial effect. Therefore, an inductive therapy by anti-CD4 in combination with conventional drug therapy is under consideration.

The antibody accumulated at the site of inflamed joints as could be demonstrated by 99m-Tc-labelled mAb. Fig.2 shows the activity accumulating in the large joints of an RA patient during the time period of 24 hours after administration. More than 10% of the total activity was detected in the joints. Affected digital joints were recognized earlier by virtue of this antibody than by conventional bone scans (12). The

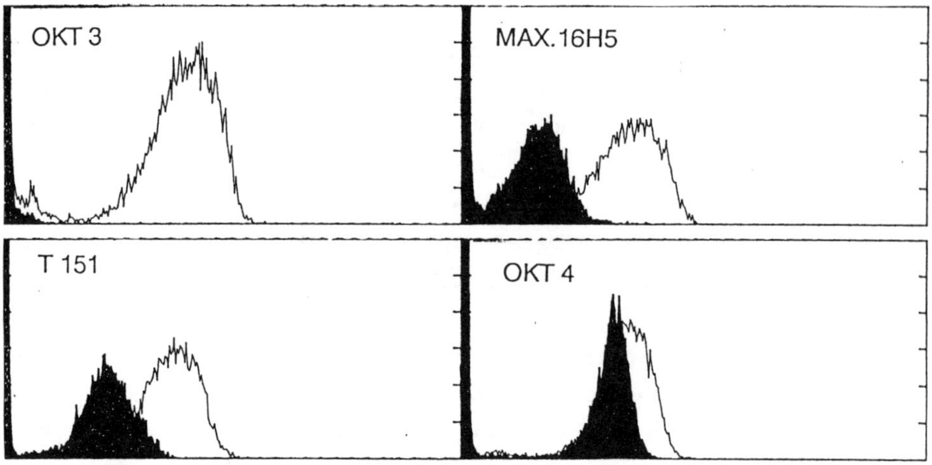

Figure 1. Differences in CD4 modulation by different mAbs. Peripheral human T cells were incubated overnight with 10μg/ml anti-CD4 (16H5, T151, OKT4) and the remaining antibody-coat was detected by an FITC-labelled goat-anti-mouse-immunoglobulin antibody (black curves). For comparison, total modulation was demonstrated for CD3 by the anti-CD3 mAb OKT3. White curves show controls that were incubated with medium and stained with anti-CD4 immediately before cytofluorometric analysis.

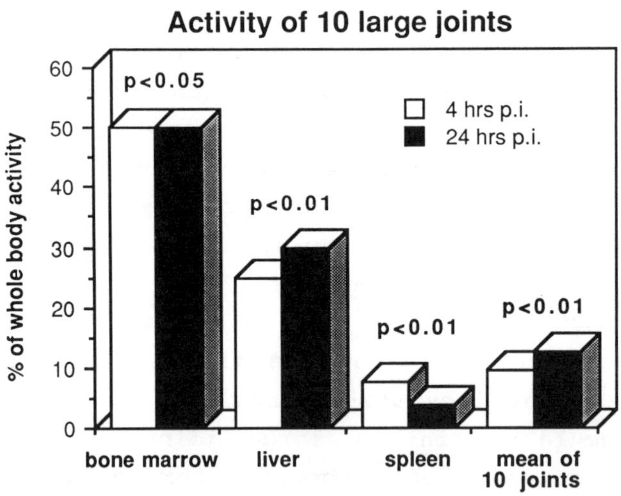

Figure 2. Activity distribution 4h and 24h after injection of Tc-99m-labelled MAX.16H5 as calculated from the whole body scans (mean) of 4 patients.

diagnostic value of $CD4^+$ T cell imaging for the detection of helper cell infiltrates in other inflammatory diseases is being explored. Initial data indicate a novel and promising diagnostic approach for chronic inflammatory diseases.

REFERENCES

1. Arnett, F.C., Edworthy, S.M., Bloch, D.A., McShane, D.J., Fries, J.F., Cooper, N.S., Healey, L.A., Kaplan, S.R. et al. (1988) Arthritis Rheum 31, 315-324
2. Emmrich, F. (1987) DMW 112, 194-198
3. Schwarz, A., Steinsträsser, A. (1987) J. Nucl. Med. 28. 721-726
4. Waldmann, H., Hale, G., Clark, M., Cobbold, S., Benjamin, R., Friend, P., Bindon, C., Dyer, M., Qin, S., Bruggemann, M. and Tighe, H. Monoclonal Antibodies for Immunosuppression. In: Monoclonal antibodies in therapy. Ed: H. Waldmann, Karger 1988, Basel p. 16-30
5. Benjamin, R.J., and Waldmann, H. (1986) Nature 320, 449-451
6. Herzog, C.H., Walker, C.H., Pichler, W., Aeschlimann, A., Wassmer P., Stockinger Knapp, W., Rieber, P. and Müller, W. (1987) Lancet II: 1461-1462
7. Emmrich, F., Lüke, G., Potocnik, A., Hunsmann, G. and Repke, H. (submitted)
8. Horneff, G., Burmester, G.R., Emmrich, F. and Kalden J.R. (submitted)
9. Qin, S., Cobbold, S., Tighe, H., Benjamin, R. and Waldmann, H. (1987) Eur. J. Immunol. 17, 1159-1165
10. Gutstein, N.L. and Wofsy, D. (1986) J. Immunol. 137, 3414-3419
11. Horneff, G., Winkler, T., Kalden, J.R., Emmrich, F. and Burmester, G.R. (submitted)
12. Becker, W., Emmrich, F., Horneff, G., Burmester, G., Seiler, G., Schwarz, A., Kalden, J.R. and Wolf, F. Eur. J. Nucl. Med. (in press)

Table I

THE BENEFIT OF ANTI-CD4 THERAPY IN PATIENTS WITH RHEUMATOID ARTHRITIS

	S.V.	H.R.I.	H.R.II	D.C.	F.H.
CB	+	–	+	+	(+)
ESR	77	0	79	45	0
CRP	87	0	95	50	0
RF	50	0	95	–	0
$CD4^+$ cells/μl	310	236	237	601	1284
0 d	11	11	18	19	138
+1 d	53	53	207	368	289
+14 d	176	176	608	299	995

CB, clinical benefit (summary); ESR, erythrocyte sedimentation rate; CRP, C-reactive protein; RF, rheumatoid factor (Latex); % of reduction after therapy at day 7
(+ significant, (+) in question, no benefit)

AAS 32
Drugs in Inflammation

MODULATION OF SPLENIC LYMPHOCYTE ACTIVITIES BY A NEW HYPOXANTHINE DERIVATIVE (ST 789) IN IMMUNOSUPPRESSED MICE

V. Ruggiero, C. Albertoni, S. Manganello, P. Foresta, E. Arrigoni Martelli

Research & Development, Dept. of Immunology and Microbiology - Sigma Tau, Pomezia, Italy.

SUMMARY:
Splenic lymphocytes of experimentally-immunosuppressed mice of different age (10 weeks and 6 months) were studied to evaluate their functional response following subcutaneous and intraperitoneal treatment with the hypoxanthine derivative N-α-5-(1,6-dihydro-6-oxo-9-purinyl)pentyloxy-carbonyl-L-arginine (ST 789). Experimental immunosuppression was carried out by injecting hybrid $B_6D_2F_1$ mice with a single dose of cyclophosphamide (100 mg/kg, i.p.) 2 hours prior to treatment with ST 789. In the young, we found that ST 789 markedly restored the splenocyte proliferative response, assessed as total amount of 3H-thymidine incorporated by mitogen-stimulated cells. In the adult, however, the ST 789-induced recovery was less pronounced. Finally, the effects of ST 789 treatment on Con A-induced IL-2 production by splenocytes were studied in normal and immunosuppressed mice of 10 weeks.

INTRODUCTION

The purine-nucleoside cycles are known to play an important role in T-lymphocyte populations. In fact, biochemical defects in purine nucleoside pathways resulting in immunological abnormalities in T-lymphocytes such as ADA deficiency and PNP deficiency were first discovered by Giblett in the early 70's (Giblett et al., 1972; Giblett et al., 1975). A role for both inosine and hypoxanthine derivatives in the regulation of several T cell functions has recently been postulated (Hadden et al., 1983). Although a sizable amount of evidence suggests a pivotal role for both inosine and hypoxanthine in the regulation of T cell proliferation and differentiation, the molecular mechanisms underlying such activities have not yet been fully elucidated.

In the early 80's, interesting results obtained by different groups (Cornaglia-Ferraris et al., 1982; Hadden et al., 1983) involved in the study of the immunomodulatory properties of some hypoxanthine and inosine derivatives paved the way for the synthesis of a new family of hypoxanthine derivatives. These derivatives are characterized by an aminoacid group joined to the N9-position of the purine ring by a pentyloxycarbonil chain. In the present report we have studied the immunomodulatory effects of a prototype drug of this family, namely N-α-5-(1,6-dihydro-6-oxo-9-purinyl) pentyloxycarbonyl-L-arginine (ST 789), formerly denominated PCF 39 (Figure 1). Our goal was to evaluate the effects of ST 789 in vivo administration on the functional activities of splenic lymphocytes from experimentally-immunosuppressed mice in comparison with those of fully immunocompetent animals.

FIGURE 1

ST 789

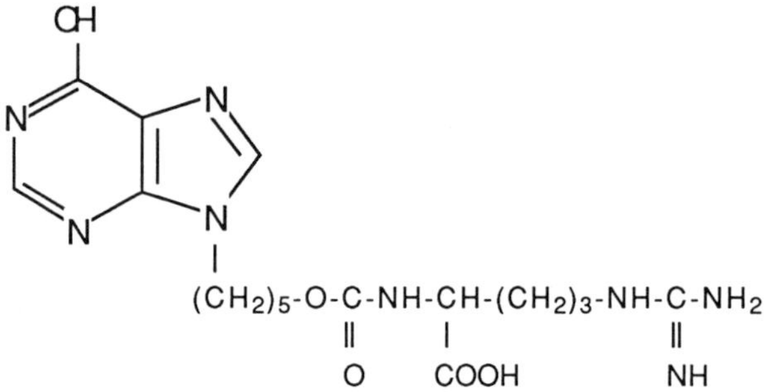

$C_{17}H_{26}N_8O_5$ M.W.= 422.44

MATERIALS AND METHODS

Tissue culture medium: RPMI-1640 supplemented with 10% heat inactivated FCS was used throughout the experiments. It was also additioned with 5×10^{-5} M 2-mercaptoethanol when culturing CTLL 2 cells.

Animals: Hybrid $B_6D_2F_1$ mice (Charles River) aged 10 weeks and 6 months were used.

Mitogens: PHA, ConA and LPS were used at 3 different concentrations (suboptimal, optimal and superoptimal conc.) as follows: 0.5-2-4 mcg/ml (PHA), 0.75-3-6 mcg/ml (ConA) and 0.5-150-500 mcg/ml (LPS).

Cyclophosphamide: Experimental immunosuppression was carried out by injecting mice with cyclophosphamide (100 mg/kg, i.p.) 2 hours before starting treatment with ST 789.

ST 789: The drug was administered by daily injection either i.p. (2-25 mg/kg) or s.c. (0.2-2 mg/kg) for 5 consecutive days.

Lymphocyte proliferation assay: Twenty four hours after the last ST 789 injection, the mice were sacrificed and their spleens were pooled (5 spleens for each experimental group) and teased. Splenocytes were then adjusted to a density of 5×10^6 cells/ml and seeded (0.1 ml/well) in a U-bottomed 96-well microtiter plate. Triplicate samples were incubated for 48 h at 37°C in a 5% CO_2 incubator with either PHA or ConA or LPS as indicated above (see Mitogens).

The cells were then labeled by adding 0.5 µCi/well of ^{3}H-TdR, incubated for 18 h, harvested onto glass fibre filters and finally placed in a β-counter (Packard). The results were evaluated by calculating the area under curve (AUC) obtained by plotting the cpm values versus the 3 different mitogen concentrations. In order to have a "stimulation index", we have also determined the ratio (Q) between AUCs of treated and control groups. With this kind of analysis, values of $Q>1$ indicate a stimulating action, whereas values <1 reflect an inhibiting action. Obviously, values equal to 1 indicate a lack of effects.

IL-2 production assay: In order to promote IL-2 production, splenocytes (5×10^6 cells/well in a 24-well plate) were cultured with ConA (5 mcg/ml) for 48 h at 37°C. Cell-free supernatants were then collected and assayed for IL-2 activity. IL-2 assay was performed by using a murine IL 2-dependent T cell line (CTLL-2) according to a standard published procedure (Hamblin et al., 1987).

RESULTS

Effects of ST 789 on splenocyte proliferation in young (Table I, II) and adult (Table III) cyclophosphamide-immunosuppressed mice: Splenocytes from young immunodepressed mice showed a drastic reduction of ConA-induced proliferation with Q values ranging from 0.24 to 0.51. It can be seen that intraperitoneal treatment with ST 789 noticeably increased the splenocyte proliferative response at the dose of 25 mg/kg/day (Q= 1.80). Similar results were otained with ST 789 administered subcutaneously (Q= 1.88).

The PHA-induced proliferation of splenocyte from young immunosuppressed mice was not so markedly impaired as seen with ConA (Q ranging from 0.44 to 0.74). In this case ST 789 was able to almost fully restore the splenocyte proliferation when injected intraperitoneally at the dose of 25 mg/kg/day (Q= 2.16), while being completely ineffective when administered subcutaneously.

Finally, when splenocytes from young immunosuppressed mice were stimulated with LPS, it was found a severe impairment in their proliferation (Q= 0.19). ST 789 significantly increased the splenocyte proliferative response when injected i.p. both at 2 mg/kg/day and at 25 mg/kg/day (Q= 1.78 and 1.74, respectively); furthermore, also the subcutaneous administration (2 mg/kg/day) turned out to be very effective (Q= 2.91).

Mice aged 6 months were used to assess whether ST 789 was able to restore the splenocyte proliferative response also in adult immunosuppressed mice. It can be seen (Table III) that ConA-induced proliferation of splenocytes from immunosuppressed mice was diminished giving a Q value of 0.43. A partial recovery of splenocyte proliferative response was obtained by administering ST 789 (2 mg/kg/day) either by s.c. or i.p. injection (Q= 1.26 and 1.32, respectively). Unespectedly, intraperitoneal administration of ST 789 at the dose of 25 mg/kg/day turned out to be ineffective.

Table I Mitogen-induced splenocyte proliferation of $B_6D_2F_1$ mice aged 10 weeks after subcutaneous treatment with ST 789. Evaluation of the area under curve (AUC) and of relevant stimulation index (Q).

Treatment	Con A AUC* (x10^{-3})	Con A Q*	PHA AUC* (x10^{-3})	PHA Q*	LPS AUC* (x10^{-5})	LPS Q*
Control	n.d.		118 (109-126)		n.d.	
Control Immunosup.			62 (53-71)	0.52○ (0.42-0.65)		
ST 789 (0.2 mg/kg)△			67 (6I-73)	1.08● (0.86-1.38)		
Control	800 (747-823)		258 (250-266)		153 (149-157)	
Control Immunosup.	289 (279-299)	0.36○ (0.34-0.40)	191 (183-198)	0.74○ (0.69-0.80)	29 (26-31)	0.19○ (0.17-0.21)
ST 789 (2 mg/kg)△	543 (524-561)	1.88● (1.75-2.01)	195 (184-207)	1.02● (0.93-1.13)	85 (80-90)	2.91● (2.53-3.37)

△ : ST 789 was administered by daily injection for 5 consecutive days to mice experimentally immunosuppressed with cyclophosphamide (100 mg/kg, i.p.) 2 hours before starting ST 789 treatment.
* : The range of AUC and Q variation is reported in brackets
○ : Q value calculated with respect to the normal control
● : Q value calculated with respect to the immunosuppressed control
n.d.= not determined

Table II Mitogen-induced splenocyte proliferation of $B_6D_2F_1$ mice aged 10 weeks after intraperitoneal treatment with ST 789. Evaluation of the area under curve (AUC) and of relevant stimulation index (Q).

Treatment	Con A AUC* (x10^{-3})	Con A Q*	PHA AUC* (x10^{-3})	PHA Q*	LPS AUC* (x10^{-5})	LPS Q*
Control	625 (610-640)		n.d.		153 (149-157)	
Control Immunosup.	317 (305-329)	0.51○ (0.48-0.54)			29 (26-31)	0.19○ (0.17-0.21)
ST 789 (2 mg/kg)△	363 (352-374)	1.15● (1.07-1.23)			52 (46-57)	1.78● (1.48-2.14)
Control	772 (735-810)		106 (100-112)		153 (149-157)	
Control Immunosup.	182 (167-197)	0.24○ (0.21-0.27)	46 (44-48)	0.44○ (0.39-0.48)	29 (26-31)	0.19○ (0.17-0.21)
ST 789 (25 mg/kg)△	330 (313-346)	1.80● (1.59-2.06)	100 (96-104)	2.16● (1.96-2.37)	50 (46-54)	1.74● (1.48-2.05)

△ : ST 789 was administered by daily injection for 5 consecutive days to mice experimentally immunosuppressed with cyclophosphamide (100 mg/kg, i.p.) 2 hours before starting ST 789 treatment.
* : The range of AUC and Q variation is reported in brackets
○ : Q value calculated with respect to the normal control
● : Q value calculated with respect to the immunosuppressed control
n.d.= not determined

Effects of ST 789 on IL-2 production in young cyclophosphamide-immunosuppressed mice (Table IV): In this study the ST 789 treatment of fully immunocompetent mice was also included and the relevant data indicate that the substance, at the dose of 25 mg/kg/day i.p., induced a significant increase in IL-2 production ($p \leq 0.05$).
Conversely, the significant decrease ($p \leq 0.05$) of IL-2 production in immunosuppressed mice was only partially restored following ST 789 treatment.

DISCUSSION

In a previous study (Foresta et al., 1988) we have shown that in vivo injections of ST 789 are able to exert marked protective effects in mice immunodepressed with cyclophosphamide and experimentally infected with several microbial pathogens. The results of this study also suggested that ST 789 could exert its effects by modulating the host immune system. In the present report we addressed ourselves at evaluating whether ST 789 might be effective in restoring the mitogen-induced proliferative response of lymphocytes from immunosuppressed mice. To this end, splenic lymphocytes of cyclophosphamide-immunosuppressed mice of different age (10 weeks and 6 months) were studied to evaluate their functional response after subcutaneous and intraperitoneal treatment with ST 789. In young mice (Tables I and II), we found that ST 789 markedly restored the proliferation of splenocytes. This recovery was most pronounced when LPS was used to induce the splenocyte proliferative response, but it was also noticed when other mitogens such as PHA and ConA were used. After assessing the immunopotentiating effect of ST 789 on splenocyte proliferation, we examined whether such activity could partially or completely be attributed to an enhanced IL-2 production.
In fully immunocompetent young mice, actually, we found (Table IV) that treatment with ST 789 significantly increased IL-2 production. Conversely, the significant decrease of IL-2 production in immunosuppressed mice was only partially restored following ST 789 treatment. However it must be pointed out that assays of IL-2 activity were performed after stimulating the splenocytes with ConA (an IL-2 inducer) only for 48 hours.

Table III ConA-induced splenocyte proliferation of $B_6D_2F_1$ mice aged 6 months after treatment with ST 789. Evaluation of the area under curve (AUC) and of relevant stimulation index (Q).

Treatment	ConA AUC* ($x10^{-3}$)	ConA Q*
Control	384 (346-422)	
Control Immunosup.	165 (154-176)	0.43○ (0.36-0.51)
ST 789 (2 mg/kg s.c.)△	207 (198-217)	1.26● (1.13-1.41)
ST 789 (2 mg/kg i.p.)△	217 (199-236)	1.32● (1.13-1.54)
ST 789 (25 mg/kg i.p.)△	165 (152-177)	1.00● (0.86-1.15)

△: ST 789 was administered by daily injection for 5 consecutive days to mice experimentally immunosuppressed with cyclophosphamide (100 mg /kg, i.p.) 2 hours before starting ST 789 treatment.
*: The range of AUC and Q variation is reported in brackets
○: Q value calculated with respect to the normal control
●: Q value calculated with respect to the immunosuppressed control

Table IV Effects of treatment with ST 789 on ConA-induced IL 2 production by splenocytes from $B_6D_2F_1$ mice aged 10 weeks.

	IL 2 (U/ml)
Control	27.10±2.13
ST 789 (25 mg/kg i.p.)[a]	39.75±4.62▲
Control Immunosup.	19.02±2.01▲
ST 789 (25 mg/kg i.p.)[b]	24.48±6.68

ST 789 was administered by daily injection for 5 consecutive days either to control mice (a) or to cyclophosphamide-immunosuppresed mice (b). At 24h after last ST 789 treatment, splenocytes from sacrificed mice (4 animals per group) were cultured 48h in the presence of ConA (5 mcg/ml). After incubation, cell-free supernatants were assayed for IL 2 activity.
Student's "t" test (ST 789 vs. control, and control immunosup. vs. control): ▲ $p<0.05$

From a kinetic standpoint, we do not yet know whether this time window is the most convenient to make adequate comparisons. In fact, it might very well be that ST 789 could actively restore IL-2 production either at earlier or later times. Experiments now in progress in our laboratories are trying to answer these questions.

In the present report, we also undertook preliminary experiments in an attempt to assess whether ST 789 might restore the splenocyte proliferative response also in adult immunosuppressed mice. Initial findings (Table III) indicate that, at least in the case of ConA-induced proliferation, the ST 789-induced recovery is less pronounced than previously found in young mice. Presently, experiments are being performed in our laboratories to test both the PHA- and LPS-induced lymphocyte proliferation and the ConA-induced IL-2 production in adult immunosuppressed mice treated with ST 789 in order to further clarify the role of such hypoxanthine derivative in these experimental models.

Acknowledgements: the skilful secretarial assistance of Mrs. L. Anconitano is gratefully acknowledged.

REFERENCES

Cornaglia-Ferraris, P., (1985) Immunomodulatory properties of N-9 substituted purines, Therapeutika, 2, 329.

Foresta, P., Albertoni, C., Marconi, A., Ramacci, M.T., and De Simone, C., (1988) Evaluation of the protective effect of a new hypoxanthine derivative (PCF 39) against experimental infections in cyclophosphamide immunocompromised mice, Pharm. Res. Com., 20, Suppplement 2, 155.

Giblett, E.R., Anderson, J.E., Cohen, F., Pollara, B., and Meuwissen, H.J., (1972) Adenosine-deaminase deficiency in two patients with severely impaired cellular immunity, Lancet, 2, 1067.

Giblett, E.R., Amman, A.J., Wara, D.W., Sandman, R., and Diamond, L.K., (1975) Nucleoside-phosphorylase deficiency in a child with severely defective T cell immunity and normal B cell immunity, Lancet, 1, 1010.

Hadden, J.W., Cornaglia-Ferraris, P. and Coffey, R.G., (1983) Purine analogs as immunomodulators. In: Progress in Immunology (Y. Yamamura and T. Tada, Eds), Academic Press, Orlando, vol. 5, 1393.

Hamblin, A.S., and O'Garra, A., (1987) Assays for interleukins and other related factors. In: Lymphocytes, a practical approach (G.G.B. Klaus, Eds), IRL Press, Washington, 209.

AAS 32
Drugs in Inflammation

THE NEWLY DEVELOPED NEUTROPHIL OXIDATIVE BURST ANTAGONIST APOCYNIN INHIBITS JOINT-SWELLING IN RAT COLLAGEN ARTHRITIS

Bert A. 't Hart[1], Nicolaas P.M. Bakker[1], Rudi P. Labadie[2] and Jos M. Simons[2]

1: Dept. chronic and infectious diseases, ITRI-TNO, P.O. Box 5815, 2280 HV Rijswijk, 2) Dept. Pharmacognosy, faculty of Pharmacy, University of Utrecht.

SUMMARY: Methylated catechols like apocynin selectively inhibits neutrophil superoxide production without significant side-effects. When rats were treated orally with low doses of apocynin the severity of collagen-induced arthritis was significantly reduced, pointing at a role of oxyradicals in the induction of this disease.

INTRODUCTION

Stimulated neutrophils can reduce free molecular oxygen to superoxide anion (S.O.) with a NADPH-dependent oxido-reductase in their membrane (Bellavite, 1988). The activation of the enzyme involves coupling of cytosolic proteins with membrane-bound subunits via S-S bridges (Akard et al., 1988). Together with released proteases, S.O.-derived reactive oxygen species (R.O.S.) form the tissue-destructive equipment of neutrophils, such as in arthritic joints (Weiss et al., 1989). The assembly can be prevented in a highly specific manner with simple methylated catechols, such as apocynin (Simons et al., 1990). In this study we describe the mechanism of this inhibition. Furthermore, we have tested the anti-arthritic activity of apocynin in rat collagen-induced arthritis (CIA), a disease in which neutrophils are actively involved (Schrier et al.).

MATERIALS AND METHODS

Neutrophil oxyradicals: Neutrophils were stimulated with the phorbol ester PMA (10 ng/ml) or with zymosan opsonized in human serum (STZ, 1.2 mg/ml). R.O.S. production was monitored in a chemiluminescence (CL) assay with lucigenin (MPO-independent R.O.S.) or luminol (MPO-dependent R.O.S.). Details were as described (Simons et al., 1990). MPO activity was determined as described ('t Hart et al., 1990a). In this study the catechol protocatechuic acid and the two methylated catechols apocynin and vanillic acid were used.

Arthritis induction: Male WAG/RIJ rats (10-12 weeks of age, mean weight about 250 g) were immunized with bovine type II collagen (B-CII) in complete Freunds adjuvant as described ('t Hart et al., 1990c). The thickness of the ankles of both hind-paws was measured (in mm) and summarized. The arthritic score was calculated by subtracting the summarized hind-ankle thickness of age-matched non-immunized animals. Daily during the indicated period 500 ul of 0.09 (final 0.3 ug/ml) or 2.4 mg (final 8 ug/ml) apocynin per ml 96% ethanol was mixed with 150 ml of fresh acidified drinking water.

ELISA: Blood samples taken by orbita punction were allowed to coagulate for 1 hour at 37°C. The presence of B-CII-specific IgG antibodies in the sera was determined with ELISA as described ('t Hart et al, 1990c).

RESULTS

Effect on neutrophil R.O.S. production: Table I shows the effect of apocynin on MPO-independent (CL_{luc}) as well as MPO-dependent (CL_{lum}) R.O.S. production. STZ-induced-, but not PMA-induced CL_{luc} was decreased in a dose-dependent manner. In contrast STZ- as well as PMA-induced CL_{lum} was inhibited. Neutrophils stimulated with STZ generate R.O.S. and release MPO and proteases.

table I: Effect of apocynin on neutrophil R.O.S. production.

apocynin	PMA-CL_{luc}	STZ-CL_{luc}	PMA-CL_{lum}	STZ-CL_{lum}
0	100%	100%	100%	100%
0.2 ug/ml	109%	90%	73%	85%
0.9 ug/ml	112%	51%	48%	53%
3.8 ug/ml	145%	26%	24%	24%
15.0 ug/ml	178%	15%	20%	10%

table II: MPO dependent metabolic activation

a) % PMA-induced CL_{luc}

	- HRPO		+ 17uM HRPO	
	I	II	I	II
apocynin (5 ug/ml)	273	196	49	73
vanillic acid (25 ug/ml)	110	189	37	56
protocatechuic acid (5 ug/ml)	63	53	55	58

b) % CL_{luc}

	STZ		PMA	
	I	II	I	II
vanillic acid (40 ug/ml)	95	99	92	111
protocatechuic acid (6 ug/ml)	27	53	49	49

In contrast, PMA-stimulated neutrophils produce also R.O.S. but release only little MPO ('t Hart et al, 1990a). For the inhibitory effect of apocynin on CL_{luc} release of MPO is therefore obligatory. This was proven in two experiments. Table IIa shows that addition of horse radish peroxidase (HRPO) causes inhibition of PMA-induced CL_{luc} by apocynin and vanillic acid. Furthermore, table IIb shows that the catechol protocatechuic acid but not the methylated catechol vanillic acid inhibits PMA- and STZ-induced CL_{luc} by MPO-deficient rat alveolar macrophages. At increasing concentrations apocynin inhibits MPO activity which explains the stimulation of PMA-induced CL_{luc}, because MPO-dependent R.O.S. are involved in termination of NADPH oxido-reductase activity (Jandl et al., 1977).

Effect of apocynin on rat CIA: Rats were immunized with B-CII in CFA.

Treatment with the indicated doses of apocynin via the drinking water was started at day 8 after immunization, that is just before the onset of joint-swelling, and continued till day 22.

table III: effect of apocynin on B-CII-specific IgG production

apocynin (µg/ml)	Abs. at 405 (O.D.± SEM)		
	1/100	1/400	1/1600
0	823 ± 18	642 ± 71	252 ± 69
0.3	908 ± 92	503 ± 119	149 ± 38
8.0	868 ± 60	549 ± 120	190 ± 49

Fig. 1 shows that the lowest apocynin dose completely inhibited joint-swelling. At increasing concentrations the effect was reduced. This is likely due to fact that apocynin inhibits its own metabolic activation by the previously discussed inhibition of MPO. Because IgG antibodies to the inciting antigen can induce CIA (table III: B-CII-specific antibodies) (Stuart et al., 1982) the serum-levels of B-CII-specific IgG determined immediately after termination of the apocynin-treatment. Table III shows no suppressive effect of apocynin.

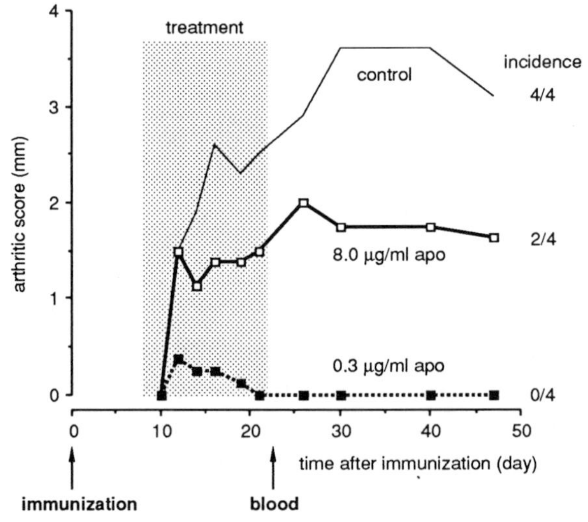

Fig.1: Effect of apocynin on rat CIA

DISCUSSION

Recently a new activity of the methylated catechol apocynin and some structurally related molecules was found, namely the selective inhibition of neutrophil R.O.S. production. The working mechanism proved to involve peroxidase-dependent metabolic activation after which reaction products prevent assembly of the S.O.-generating oxido-reductase. The reaction products were not identified, but quinone-methides and orthoquinones can be formed. The inhibitory effect of apocynin is limited to R.O.S. production because phagocytosis and degranulation are not affected (not shown) only minor side-effects to non-phagocytosing cells such as lymphocytes were found, such as on mitogen-induced proliferation in vitro, and on antibody production in vivo.

Taking this selectivity into account, the observed inhibition of CIA in rats treated with apocynin point at an important role of R.O.S. in the pathogenesis of this disease. The role of R.O.S. in cartilage destruction and the development of autoimmunity is subject of our present research.

REFERENCES:

Akard, L.P., English, D., and Gabig, T.G. (1988) Rapid deactivation of NADPH oxidase in neutrophils. Blood 72, 322-327.

Bellavite, P. (1988) The superoxide-forming enzymatic system of phagocytes. Free Radical Biol. Med. 4, 225-261.

Jandl, B.S., Andre-Schwartz, J., Borges-Dubois, L., Kipnes, R.S., McMurrich, B.J., Babior, B.S. (1977) Termination of the respiratory burst in human neutrophils. J. Clin. Invest. 61, 1176-1185.

't Hart, B.A., Ip Vai Ching T.R.A.M., van Dijk, H., and Labadie R.P. (1990a) How flavonoids inhibit the generation of luminol-dependent chemiluminescence by activated human neutrophils. Chem. Biol. Interactions 73, 323-325.

't Hart B.A., Simons, J.M., Rijkers, G.T., Hoogvliet, J.C., van Dijk, H., and Labadie R.P. (1990b) Reaction products of 1-naphthol with reactive oxygen species prevent NADPH oxidase activation in activated human neutrophils. Free Radical Biol. Med. 8, 241-249.

't Hart, B.A., Simons, J.M., Knaan-Shanzer, S., Bakker, N.P.M., and Labadie, R.P. (1990c) Anti-arthritic activity of the recently developed neutrophil oxiradical antagonist apocynin. Free Radical Biol. Med., in press.

Schrier, D., Gilbertsen, R.B., Lesch, M., and Fantone, J. (1984) The role of neutrophils in type II collagen arthritis in rats. Am. J. Pathol. 117, 26-29.
Simons, J.M., 't Hart, B.A., Ip Vai Ching, T.R.A.M., van Dijk, H., and Labadie, R.P. (1990) Metabolic activation of natural phenols into selective oxidative burst agonists by activated human neutrophils. Free Radical Biol. Med. 8, 251- 258.
Stuart, J.M., Cremer, M.A., Townes, A.S., and Kang, A.H. (1982) Type II collagen-induced arthritis in rats. J. exp. Med. 155, 1-16.
Thompson, D., Norbeck, K., Olsson, L.I., Constatin-Teodosiu, D., van der Zee, J., and Moldeus, P. (1989) Peroxidase-catalyzed oxidation of eugenol. J. Biol. Chem. 264, 1016-1021.
Weiss, S.J. (1989) Tissue destruction by neutrophils. N. Engl. J. Med. 320, 365-375.

key words: apocynin, peroxidase, metabolic activation, oxiradicals, neutrophils, collagen-induced arthritis.

AUTO-IMMUNE SPONDYLODISCITIS ASSOCIATED WITH COLLAGEN INDUCED ARTHRITIS IN RATS: HIGH FIELD MRI FINDINGS

P Gillet[1], P Fener[1], JM Escanyé[2], P Walker[2], B Bannwarth[1], JY Jouzeau[1], E Drelon[1], J Floquet[3], P Netter[1], J Robert[2] and A Gaucher[1]

1. Departments of Pharmacology & Rheumatology, URA CNRS 1288
2. Laboratoire de Biophysique
3. Department of Pathology
Université de Nancy 1 et CHRU Nancy Brabois, F 54505 Vandoeuvre Les Nancy

SUMMARY: The spinal involvement of the tail was studied in Wistar Furth rats immunized with bovine native type II collagen. Focal caudal autoimmune spondylodiscitis occured 5 weeks after sensitization, as assessed histopathologically. High field Magnetic Resonance Imaging (MRI) was useful in depicting these caudal abnormalities that were related to juxta-diskal enthesitis. The occurrence of such inflammatory enthesopathies could serve as an experimental approach for physiopathological and therapeutical studies of spondylarthropathies.

Collagen induced arthritis (CIA) is an experimental model of chronic joint inflammation that can be induced in rodents by immunization against homologous or heterologous native type II collagen (CII). This chronic, polyarticular arthritis involves principally peripheral small and medium-sized joints, resulting from both erosive synovitis and periosteal new bone formation. Nevertheless, during CIA the vertebral skeleton is relatively untouched, except in a few reported cases of nodulation of the tail related to auto-immune spondylitis (Cremer et al., 1984).

In order to assess whether immunization against native CII induces subacute axial skeletal inflammation, we performed a high field MR imaging prospective study of the tail in arthritic and normal rats. Our results were correlated with conventional radiographs and histological evaluation.

MATERIALS AND METHODS

Immunization procedure: on day 0, 38 female Wistar Furth rats (120-150g) were injected subcutaneously with 500µg of bovine native CII (Bioetica, Lyon, France) emulsified (v/v) in Freund's incomplete adjuvant (FIA). On day 7, rats were given a booster *sc* injection of 500 µg CII+FIA. In addition, 11 naive rats served as controls. Two rats (1 arthritic and 1 naive) were sacrificed at regular intervals (days 14,21,26,33,40,47,56,

70,98,138,161) after radiological and MR procedure. In parallel one arthritic rat was studied prospectively at the same intervals to define the sequence of the evolving X ray and MR features.

Clinical and radiological evaluation: rats were regularly clinically observed for the development of CIA until sacrifice. For radiological and MR studies, the rats were anesthetized with a mixture of acepromazine and ketamine hydrochloride given *im*. On the same day as the MR study, conventional radiographs of the tail were obtained in arthritic rats and controls. The film was placed 62 cm below the X ray source (settings: 120 mA, 21 kV and 0.15 sec exposure).

High field proton MR Imaging: all studies have been performed in a Bruker Biospec BMT 100 spectrometer, with a 2.4 Tesla/40 cm bore horizontal magnet. The observation frequency for proton was 100 MHz. In order to achieve a high sensitivity/high resolution imaging, a purpose built loop gap resonator was developed (Escanyé JM et al., 1989). It consists of a singly slotted copper tube, 30 mm in diameter, 40 mm in length. While especially good sensitivity is a characteristic of the resonator design, a major drawback is resonant frequency (RF) inhomogeneity along the slot and at the cylinder extremities. Our design did not escape this default, and the large diameter (30 mm) of the coil, compared to the diameter of the rat's tail (10-15 mm) was a means of compensating for the problem. A large foam was used, in order to position the tail in the central area of the cylinder. The measured quality factor for the coil varies from more that 300 (empty) to 195 (filled maximally). Thus we have been able to obtain high quality images without any changes to the biospec gradient coil design, with a very low RF power of 20 W, and without any repetitive scanning, for a field of view of 5 cm and a slice thickness of 2 mm. The theoretical resolution of 200μm is achieved only without any motion of the animals, thus the "no repetition" scanning is very important. In this study we have performed standard spin echo images, with the T1 weighted repetition rate of 500 ms, and the T2 weighted repetition rate of 2000 ms. This point should be considered as a first step procedure, before quantitative measurement of the relaxation time T1 and T2. The images were obtained thus in 2 minutes and 8 minutes respectively.

Histopathology: after MRI and conventional radiographic study, rats were sacrificed, and the selected segment of the tails were placed in Bouin's solution for 48 h, immersed in decalcifying solution for 2-4 days, and embedded in paraffin. Sections were then cut sagitally and stained with Hematoxylin and Eosin.

RESULTS

Clinical and radiological evaluation of the arthritis: immunization against bovine native CII induced 50% arthritis in rats in our sensitization procedure. Arthritis became obvious around day 14 post-injection, with swelling and erythema in ankle or tarsal joints, and digits. The onset of vertebral involvement was delayed. It consisted of a slight focal tumefaction palpable on day 40, with contiguous mild redness lasting for 2 weeks. Then, after day 70, most of these segmentar vertebral locations of CIA were no longer detectable, excepting 2 rats with persisting nodulation of the tail. Radiologically, a notch involving the angles of the vertebral plates was detectable on day 98.

MR features of the tail with histopathological correlations:

Appearance of the normal tail in MR images: in sagittal cross section of the normal tail, the vertebrae were easily highlighted as high density structures on T1 and T2 sequences, due to strong signal generated by bone marrow. Cortical bone is of low density. Intervertebral disk appeared as an intermediate signal, with a central spot of high signal, in T2 weighted sequences, representing nucleus pulposus and its important water content (Figure 1). Periarticular soft tissues were of heterogenous intermediate density and represented an average of different tissue types, including ligamentous, muscle and fatty tissues.

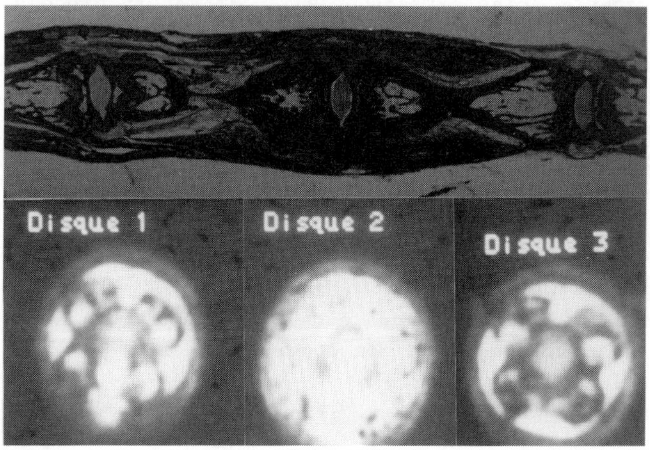

Figure 1: Segmental caudal spondylodiscitis in rat; MRI with histological correlation. **a**. sagittal section of the tail (HES x 80); three intervertebral spaces are shown: 1 and 3 are normal; in 2 note the inflammatory infiltrate in the area of attachment of the annulus fibrosus
b: MR axial scan, T2 weighted sequence (TR=2034msec/TE=34msec). marked hypersignal in the vertebral disk n°2

Inflammatory changes in the tail: between days 14-26 no evident changes were detected on MR scans. From day 33, a slightly increased signal was detected on T2 weighted sequences around the intervertebral disk, while no changes were evident on T1 weighted images. In contrast, radiographs remained normal. The T2 hypersignal intensity peaked on day 47 in foci of inflammatory lesions. It then decreased and disappeared without sequellae. Corresponding to histological evaluation, these MR features were typical of caudal auto-immune spondylodiscitis (d33-d47), associated with a peridiskal inflammatory infiltrate, predominating at the insertions of the annulus fibrosus on the vertebral plate. There were also zones of periostitis on the lateral face of vertebral bodies. These enthesitis were associated with slight bony erosions, chondroblastic proliferation and a subsequent slight cicatricial fibrosis (day 56-day 161).

Prospective study: the rat observed at regular intervals was affected by a congestive spondylodiscitis, beginning on day 47 and progressively resolving into a mild cicatricial fibrosis.

DISCUSSION

This study confirms our previous observation that WF rats, when injected with heterologous native type II collagen emulsified in FIA may develop polyarthritis and clinically subacute nodulation of the tail. Such a caudal disease is evidence of an extrasynovial inflammatory process predominating on the peridiskal ligamentous insertions. The inflammation of theses entheses is a central feature of the vertebral involvement in this animal model and in human spondylarthritides. We have therefore previously suggested that CIA could be an experimental model of spondylarthropathy (Gillet et al., 1989).

Evaluation of the severity of joint damage is necessary in order to assess the efficacy of anti-arthritic treatments during experimental arthritis, but radiographic assessment shows diagnostically characteristic changes only late in the arthritic process. Moreover, radiography is not sensitive enough to subtle changes either in disease activity or in disease progression or improvement. On the other hand, MRI has many features that could make it ideal for joint imaging, but little has been published about its application to the experimental arthritis.

The only full of MRI study of animal models of arthritis used is antigen induced arthritis in the rabbit knee (Checkley et al., 1989) and the rat adjuvant model (Terrier et al., 1985). Nevertheless, the small size of these models and the resolution of the instrument limit the ability to distinguish specific changes in the joints. We thus employed an experimental model of auto-immune caudal spondylodiscitis in the rat, with the aid of a purpose built loop gap resonator for the tail. High field MRI allows tissue discrimination between the different anatomical structures, both within and near intervertebral disks of the tail. Furthermore MRI clearly revealed the long T2 tissues associated with the juxta-diskal inflammation with a good histological correlation, and allows the prediction of time course in the development of this caudal disease.

CONCLUSION: high field MR imaging seems likely to be of value in the early, non invasive diagnosis of subacute experimental caudal auto-immune spondylodiscitis in rats immunized against native type II collagen. Further studies are required to assess the accuracy of MRI in quantitating the inflammatory process. Such a quantification of magnetic parameters, like T1 relaxation time, could allow non invasive follow up studies in arthritic animals receiving different anti-inflammatory drugs. This is the object of our current investigations.

REFERENCES

Checkley,D., Johnstone,D., Taylor,K. and Waterton,JC. (1989) High resolution NMR imaging of an antigen induced arthritis in the rabbit knee. *Magnetic Resonance in Medicine*, **11**:21-235

Cremer,MA., Townes,AS. and Wang,AM. (1984) Collagen induced arthritis in rodents. A review of clinical, histological and immunological features. *The Ryumachi*, **24**:45-56

Escanyé,J.M., Drelon,E., Robin-Lherbier,B., Jouzeau,J.Y., Walker, P.M., Netter,P. and Gaucher,A. (1989) Collagen induced arthritis in rats: High resolution MRI findings. *Europ J Nucl Med*, **15**:564

Gillet,P., Bannwarth,B., Charrrière,G., Leroux,P., Fener,P., Hartmann,D.J., Netter,P., Péré,P. and Gaucher,A.(1989) Studies on type II collagen induced arthritis : an experimental model of peripheral and axial enthesopathy *J Rheumatol*, **16**:721-728

Terrier,F., Hricak,H., Revel,D., Alpers,CE., Reinhold,CE., Levine,J. and Genant,HK. (1985) Magnetic resonance imaging and spectroscopy of the periarticular inflammatory soft tissue changes in experimental arthritis of the rat. *Invest Radiol*, **20**:813-823

AAS 32
Drugs in Inflammation

INFLUENCE OF MURAMYL DIPEPTIDE ON ESTABLISHED EXPERIMENTAL ARTHRITIS IN RATS

JY. Jouzeau[1], E. Drelon[1], P. Gillet[1], B. Bannwarth[1], P. Fener[1], G. Charrière[2], E. Payan[1], L. Chauvelot-Moachon[3], AM. Batt[4], J. Floquet[1], P. Netter[1] and A. Gaucher[1]

1. *Departments of Pharmacology & Rheumatology, URA CNRS 1288, F 54511 Nancy*
2. *Centre de Radio-analyse, Institut Pasteur, URA CNRS 602 F 69366 Lyon*
3. *Department of Pharmacology, URA CNRS 595 Hôpital Cochin, F 75674 Paris*
4. *Centre du Médicament, URA CNRS 597 F 54000 Nancy*

SUMMARY: The effects of MDP, a potent inducer of cytokines, were studied in four batches of Wistar Furth rats with established experimental arthritis. Arthritic rats were given a daily *sc* injection of 10, 100, 200 or 400 μg MDP respectively. Muramyl dipeptide increased the severity of clinical events in a dose-dependent manner, with the exception of the 10 μg dose which was ineffective. The levels of anti-collagen antibodies were not however significantly enhanced by MDP. Radiological lesions and histological changes were maximal at high dosage regimens. Paradoxically, the acute phase reactive $\alpha 1$ glycoprotein was little affected by MDP treatment.

Muramyl dipeptide (MDP), is the minimal chemical structure of bacterial cell-wall peptidoglycans required for immuno-adjuvanticity. MDP stimulates macrophages to produce and release various soluble factors such as interleukin 1 (IL1) and prostaglandin E_2. These factors appear to play a key role as mediators or as modulators of the different stages of inflammation. The increase of IL1 synthesis has further been proposed to be one of the major mechanisms of adjuvanticity. On the other hand, MDP exerts ambivalent immunomodulatory activities, increasing or decreasing humoral and cellular responses, depending upon the experimental conditions used. In the same manner, MDP is able under special conditions to be arthritogenic in some strains of rats (Nagao et al., 1980; Zidek et al., 1982), while it exhibited at some doses an anti-inflammatory activity.

The aim of the present study, was to investigate the effect of various doses of MDP on the course of an established experimental arthritis model in rats.

MATERIALS AND METHODS

Animals and reagents: inbred female Wistar-Furth rats (n=58) weighing 110-120g were kept in group of 5 in plastic cages with free access to water and standard laboratory food. On day 0, rats were injected intradermally with 80 μg human native type II collagen (CII) and 0.2 mg of MDP both emulsified *v/v* in Freund's incomplete adjuvant (FIA). On day 8, animals were given a booster injection of 15 μg CII emulsified with FIA (Gillet et al., 1989). Rats were sacrificed under anaesthesia by cardiac exsanguination on day 35.

MDP treatment: on day 21, rats with polyarthritis (n=35) were assessed on the three non-injected legs, and were randomly assigned to 5 groups. Non arthritic rats were not further studied. The treatment was administered *sc* in the right flank after local asepsis. MDP batches received daily 10μg, 100μg, 200μg and 400μg respectively in 0.25ml of 9% saline from day 21 to day 28. The control batch received in the same manner the vehicle only (9% saline).

Clinical severity of arthritis: rats were examined daily by the same investigator who was blind to the treatment. The scoring system was based on severity and extent of erythema and swelling of the 3 uninjected paws yielding a maximal score of 12 per animal.

Hindpaw volume was regularly assessed using a mercury plethysmograph (ΔV3 model, Ugo Basile Milan). The results were expressed as the mean extent of the paw edema with the difference against initial value for each rat : $\Delta \text{ ml} = \text{Volume}_{\text{day observed}} - \text{Volume}_{\text{day 21}}$

Serological procedures: blood samples were drawn by veinipuncture at the base of the tail before sensitization and on days 21 and 28 and by cardiac puncture just before sacrifice (day 35). Sera were swiftly prepared and stored at -20°C until assay. Humoral response to collagen was quantified by a solid phase radio-immunoassay (Charrière et al., 1985). Alpha-1 acid glycoprotein (α1GP) quantitation was measured by rocket immunoelectrophoresis.

Radiographic evaluation was performed after sacrifice, on the sectioned left hindpaws. Calcaneal new bone formation, metatarsophalangeal erosions, tarsal and tibiotarsal changes were graded 0 (normal) to 3 (severe). Results were recorded for each animal as the total of the radiological finding scores.

Histological assessment: knees and ankles were sliced sagitally and stained with HES. Three features were assessed: cartilage loss, bony erosions, and pannus formation. A grade 0-5 was assigned to each parameter (0: no sign, 5: severe changes).

Statistical analysis: batches were compared using an *Anova* test and *Student's t* test for quantitative parameters and the non-parametric *Mann-*

Whitney's U test for semi-quantitative variables (arthritic index, radiological score).

RESULTS

Inflammation was clinically detectable after day 15 and peripheral arthritis became obvious in 35 of the collagen-sensitized animals by day 21 (incidence = 60%). The severity of the condition peaked on day 30 with a gradual decrease thereafter. The mean arthritic index rose in a dose-dependent manner after parenteral administration of 100, 200 and 400 μg of MDP while the dose of 10 μg failed to induce any changes when compared with controls (Figure 1). In the same manner, MDP clearly increased non injected hindpaw swelling with doses ranges 100, 200 and 400 μg whilst the 10 μg dose remained ineffective.

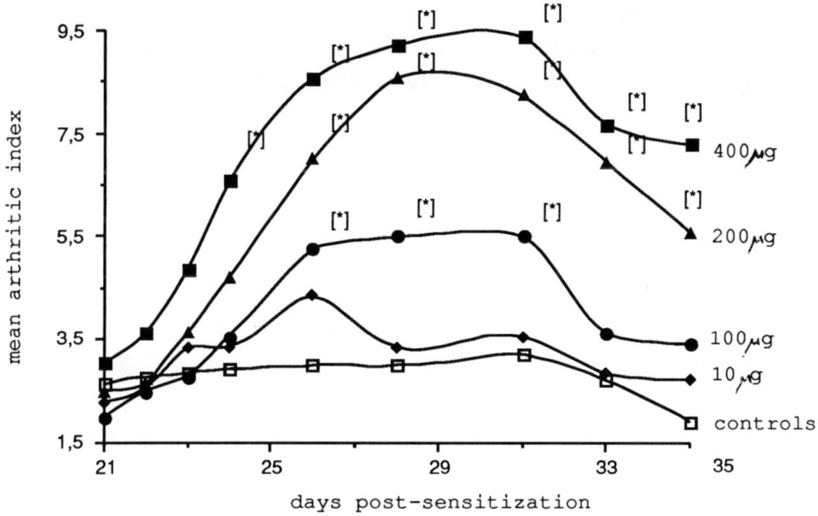

Figure 1. Time course of the severity of arthritis, expressed as the mean arthritic indices, for arthritic rats treated from day 21 to day 28 with range doses of MDP. [*] indicates significantly different when compared to controls ($p \leq 0.05$, *Mann-Withney's U* -test).

Despite of a lack of significance, the radiographical changes seemed more severe in MDP-treated groups than in the control group. Both periosteal new bone formation and juxta-articular erosions were concerned. High doses seemed however more effective in joint injury than in bony changes as reflected by a significantly higher joint erosion score in the 400 μg batch. Pathological findings corroborated the severity of these radiological features. Ankle and tarsal lesions were thus more pronounced in MDP batches, especially at high doses (200,400μg). This was reflected by enhanced cartilage loss and bony changes, and an extensive synovial pannus. In contrast femoro-tibial joint space was little affected by the arthritic process by day 35.

Wistar-Furth rats exhibited a weak physiological concentration of α1GP (0.091±0.019 g/l, n=21). The α1GP levels then showed a 9-12 fold increase in all groups as arthritis developed, before lowering to a 5-7 fold increase when the disease process subsided. The changes during the treatment period were slightly higher in MDP batches when compared with controls. However large scattering of the data led us to the exclusion of the 100μg and 200μg treated groups from any further study.

None of the Wistar-Furth rats exhibited detectable levels of antibody (IgG) in peripheral blood before sensitization. The antibody levels subsequently evolved in the same manner as polyarthritis so that all arthritic rats had high antibody titers. The rise in antibody levels was not significantly higher in MDP batches than in controls, and was unrelated to the dose of MDP. Finally, non significant correlations were found on days 21 (r=0.22), 28 (r=0.05) and 35 (r=0.11) between type II antibody titers and mean arthritic indices.

DISCUSSION

Since the clinical course of the arthritic disease was clearly increased in rats, our study confirmed the pro-inflammatory properties of MDP. Thus, repeated *sc* administration enhanced the severity of the clinical symptoms and hindpaw swelling in a dose dependent manner, with a minimal dose higher than 10μg being required (100μg in our experiment). These events are of the same date as a gradual spread of polyarthritis, as the forepaws became more frequently affected when high doses were applied.

The role of MDP in radiographical changes was not surprising as its arthritogenic potency has been well established in specific water-in-oil emulsion or in saline solution. Our results showed a disparaging effect of MDP on radiological features with marked changes on juxta-articular erosions. These findings suggested that this synthetic glycopeptide is able to enhance the previous collagen-induced arthritic lesions, as confirmed by our histological results.

The time course of anticollagen antibodies was not influenced by the *sc* administration of MDP. Hence, despite anticollagen antibodies are thought to be involved in the pathogenesis of the disease (Stuart et al., 1988), this proinflammatory property is not mediated by their enhancement. However, humoral response to collagen represents only a partial pathway, and an antigen specific T lymphokine (arthritogenic factor) might play a major role in the arthritogenicity of CII (Helfgott et al., 1985).

Although the acute phase reactive α1GP evolved in the same manner as polyarthritis, changes in serum levels appeared to be moderate in MDP treated groups. These results are quite unexpected as MDP is a potent inducer of IL1 release *in vivo* and *in vitro* (Bahr et al., 1987). However, the down-regulation of some acute phase protein has been extensively shown after continued stimulation with phlogistic agents (Wichmer et al., 1989) .

CONCLUSION: MDP is able to increase the severity of clinical, radiological and histological features when given subcutaneously during established experimental arthritis in rats. This pro-inflammatory effect is not related to an increase in anticollagen antibody levels. Surprisingly, the acute phase reactive α1GP which is inducible by IL1 and IL6, is poorly affected by MDP administration. The dosage of endogenous cytokines will be of great interest in order to assess their respective contribution during this arthritic process.

REFERENCES:

Bahr, G.M., Chedid, L. and Behbehani, K. (1987) Induction, in vivo and in vitro, of macrophage membrane interleukin 1 by adjuvant-active synthetic muramyl peptides ,*Cell Immunol*, **107**:443-454

Charrière, G., Hartman, DJ. and Ville, G. (1984) Dosage des anticorps anti-collagène par technique radio-immunologique en phase solide, *C R Soc Biol*, **178**:160-170

Gillet, P., Bannwarth, B., Charriere, G., Leroux, P., Fener, P., Netter, P., Hartmann, D.J., Pere, P. and Gaucher, A. (1989) Studies on type II collagen-induced arthritis in rats : an experimental model of peripheral and axial ossifying enthesopathy, *J Rheum*, **16** (6):721-726

Helfgott, S.M., Dynesius-Trentham, R., Brahn, E. and Trentham, D.E. (1985) An arthritogenic lymphokine in the rat, *J Exp Med*, **162**:1531-1545

Nagao, S. and Tanaka, A. (1980) Muramyl dipeptide-induced adjuvant arthritis, *Infect Immun*, **28**:624-626

Stuart, J.M., Watson, W.C. and Kang A.H. (1988) Collagen autoimmunity and arthritis, *Faseb J*, **2**:2950-2956

Zidek, Z., Masek, K. and Jiricka, Z. (1982) Arthritogenic activity of a synthetic immunoadjuvant, MDP, *Infect Immun*, **35**:674-679

Whicher, J.T., Thompson, D., Billingham, M.E.J. and Kitchen, E.A. (1989) Acute phase proteins, in Pharmacological Methods. In; The Control of Inflammation (Chang JY & Lewis AJ Eds), Alan R. Liss, Inc, New-York, pp.101-128

AAS 32
Drugs in Inflammation

SELECTIVE INHIBITION BY MAGNOSALIN AND MAGNOSHININ, COMPOUNDS FROM "SHIN-I"(FLOS MAGNOLIAE), OF ADJUVANT-INDUCED ANGIOGENESIS AND GRANULOMA FORMATION IN THE MOUSE POUCH

M. Kimura, S. Kobayashi, B. Luo and I. Kimura

Department of Chemical Pharmacology, Faculty of Pharmaceutical Sciences, Toyama Medical and Pharmaceutical University, 2630 Sugitani, Toyama 930-01, Japan

SUMMARY: Inhibitory effects of magnosalin and magnoshinin, compounds from the crude drug "Shin-i"(Flos magnoliae), on angiogenesis and pouch granuloma formation in mice induced by an adjuvant containing croton oil were investigated. The anti-chronic inflammatory effect of "shin-i" was caused by selective inhibition of angiogenesis by magnosalin and of granuloma formation by magnoshinin.

The Sino-Japanese medicine "Shin-i"(Flos magnoliae) consisting of dried flower buds of *Magnoliae salicifolia*, has been used traditionally for curing chronic rhinitis and nasosinusitis. Magnosalin and magnoshinin are isolated from "Shin-i" (Kikuchi et al., 1983), and are classed as neolignans. The present study was conducted to investigate the inhibition of adjuvant-induced angiogenesis by magnosalin and magnoshinin and to compare it with the inhibition of granuloma formation in mice.

MATERIALS AND METHODS

The amount of angiogenesis, granuloma formation and exudation of pouch fluid of granuloma was determined as previously described (Kimura et al., 1985 a, b; Kimura et al. 1986). Male ddY strain mice (6-7 week-old, 27-35 g weighing; Japan Shizuoka Laboratory Center, Hamamatsu) were used. Three ml of air was injected subcutaneously, and 0.5 ml of Freund's complete adjuvant (FCA) emulsion containing 0.1% croton oil (Nacalai, Kyoto) was injected into the air pouch formed after 24 hr. One-ml quantities of 10% (w/v) carmine dye (Merck, Darmstadt, FRG) solution containing 5% gelatin (Nacalai) were warmed at 40°C, and injected into the tail vein on the 5th day after the FCA injection. After the cadavers were cooled below 4°C for 2-3 hr, the amount of granuloma tissue and fluid in the pouch was measured by weight. The granuloma tissue was cut, suspended in 6 ml of 3 N NaOH solution at 37 °C for 20 min, neutralized with 3 ml of 36% HCl, and then centrifuged at 1,100 x g for 20 min. After the resultant supernatant was filtered through a Millipore filter (0.45 µm; Nihon Millipore Kogyo, Yonezawa), the amount of carmine in the filtrate was determined by measuring the optical density at 490 nm. Magnosalin, magnoshinin, heterotropan (a gift from Prof. T. Kikuchi, Research Institute for Wakan-Yaku [Oriental Medicines] of our University) (Fig. 1), and hydrocortisone acetate (Nacalai) were suspended in saline with 1% Avicel (Asahi Chemical Industry, Tokyo), and injected i.p. or intra-pouch 2 hr after FCA injection and subsequently once a day for 4 days.

RESULTS

Effects of magnosalin and magnoshinin intraperitoneally administered on angiogenesis, granuloma formation, and pouch exudation: Magnosalin and magnoshinin (i.p. administered) were compared for their effects on carmine content, the amount of granuloma, and the pouch exudate. Magnosalin reduced the carmine content and the pouch fluid only at 120 mg/kg, and the amount of granuloma tissue at 60 to 120 mg/kg. Magnoshinin did not reduce the carmine content even at 120 mg/kg, but it inhibited granuloma formation at 120 mg/kg and pouch fluid exudation at 60 to 120 mg/kg. The percent inhibition of granuloma formation by magnoshinin (120 mg/kg) was 1.5-fold greater than that by magnosalin. Magnoshinin was less potent by i.p. than by intra-pouch administration.

The ID_{50} values of the neolignans and hydrocortisone are estimated. The inhibitory potencies of hydrocortisone for the three inflammatory processes were above 14-fold greater by intra-pouch than by i.p. administration. Magnosalin for angiogenesis and magnoshinin for granuloma formation were 66-fold and 23-fold more potent by intra-pouch than by i.p. administration, respectively. The potency of magnoshinin against granuloma formation was above 2.5-fold greater than against angiogenesis.

Relation between the inhibitions by magnosalin, magnoshinin and hydrocortisone of angiogenesis and granuloma formation: The percent inhibition of angiogenesis was re-plotted for percent inhibition of granuloma formation by magnosalin, magnoshinin and hydrocortisone (Fig. 2). The regression lines were the least-squares lines. The regression coefficient of the inhibition of angiogenesis vs. the inhibition of granuloma formation was 1.79 for magnosalin, 1.11 for hydrocortisone and 0.61 for magnoshinin. These results indicate that magnosalin was a more selective inhibitor for angiogenesis than hydrocortisone, whereas magnoshinin was a selective inhibitor for granuloma formation.

DISCUSSION

As compared with a number of other anti-inflammatory drugs, little work has been done with agents to inhibit chronic inflammation. Such agents will not be obtained without focusing on granuloma formation in the inflammatory process, in the strict sense, followed by the angiogenesis of granuloma (Ross and Benditt, 1961; Korn, 1980). The inhibitory effect of magnosalin was selective for the angiogenesis in the sense that angiogenesis was more sensitive to the drug than was granuloma formation, and that angiogenesis was more sensitive to magnosalin than to hydrocortisone. On the other hand, magnoshinin is selective against granuloma formation because this inflammatory reaction was more sensitive to it than to hydrocortisone. Heterotropan, which resembles magnosalin in chemical structure (Kikuchi et al., 1983), did not significantly inhibit angiogenesis, suggesting that the selectivity of magnosalin needs the stereochemical specificity at the site of action.

CONCLUSION: The anti-chronic inflammatory effect of "Shin-i" is due to both selective inhibition of angiogenesis by magnosalin and of granuloma formation by magnoshinin.

Acknowledgments: This work was supported in part by the Japan Rheumatism Foundation 1989. The authors would like to thank Prof. T. Kikuchi for kindly supplying magnoshinin, magnosalin and heterotropan.

REFERENCES

Kikuchi, T., Kadota, S., Yanada, K., Tanaka, K., Watanabe, K,. Yoshizaki, M. Yokoi, T. and Shingu, T. (1983) Isolation and structure of magnosalin and magnoshinin, new neolignans from Magnolia salicifolia maxim. Chem. Pharm. Bull. 31, 1112-1114

Kimura, M., Suzuki, J. and Amemiya, K. (1985) Mouse granuloma pouch induced by Freund's complete adjuvant with croton oil. J. Pharmacobio-Dyn. 8, 393-400

Kimura, M., Suzuki, J., Yamada, T., Yoshizaki, M., Kikuchi, T., Kadota, S., and Matsuda, S. (1985) Anti-inflammatory effect of neolignans newly isolated from the crude drug "Shin-i"(Flos Magnoliae). Planta Medica 4, 291-293

Kimura, M., Amemiya, K., Yamada, T., and Suzuki, J. (1986) Quantitative method for measuring adjuvant-induced granuloma angiogenesis in insulin-treated diabetic mice. J. Pharmacobio-Dyn. 9, 442-446

Korn, J.H. (1980) Interaction of immune and connective tissue cells. Int. J. Dermatol. 19, 487-495

Ross, R., and Benditt, E.P. (1961) Wound healing and collagen formation. 1. Sequential changes in components of guinea pigs skin wounds observed in electron microscope. J. Biophys. Biochem. Cytol. 11, 677-700

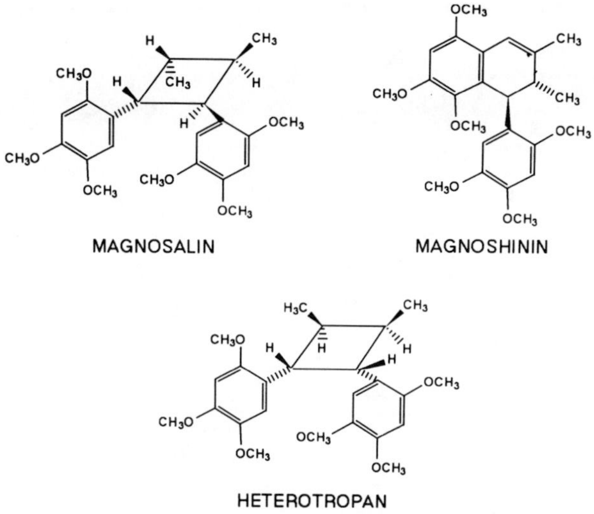

Fig. 1. Chemical structures of magnosalin, magnoshinin, and heterotropan.

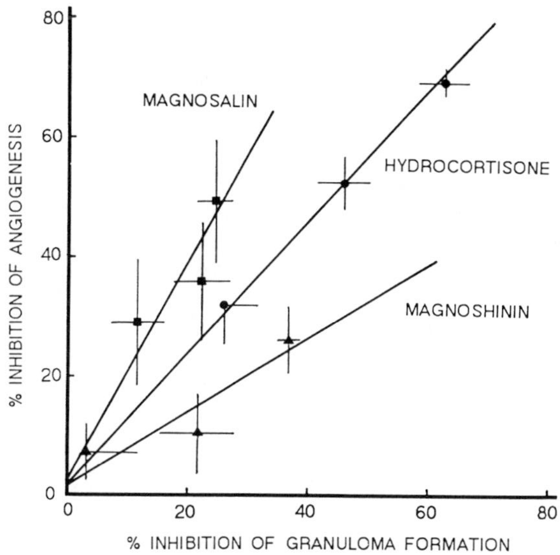

Fig. 2. Relation between the inhibition of angiogenesis and granuloma formation by magnosalin (■: 30-120 mg/kg), magnoshinin (▲: 30-120 mg/kg) and hydrocortisone (●: 3.8-15 mg/kg). These drugs were administered intraperitoneally once a day for 5 days into ddY mice injected with Freund's complete adjuvant containing 0.1% croton oil into air pouches. Absolute values of carmine content and granuloma weight without drug were 0.361 ± 0.013 mg (n=109) and 287 ± 3 mg (n=109).

Drug Modulation of Cytokine Production

AAS 32
Drugs in Inflammation

CELLULAR AND MOLECULAR MECHANISMS OF CYTOKINE NETWORKING

S. Kunkel, T. Standiford*, Stephen W. Chensue,
K. Kasahara, and R. M. Strieter*

Departments of Pathology and *Internal Medicine (Division of Pulmonary and Critical Care Medicine), The University of Michigan Medical School, 1301 Catherine Rd., Box 0602, Ann Arbor, Michigan 48109-0602

SUMMARY:

A number of scientific investigations support the theory that the coordinate expression of cytokines are paramount to the successful initiation and maintenance of inflammation. Interleukin-1 and TNF appear particularly important in that these cytokines are important as both proximal and distal mediators of disease. The importance of IL-1 and TNF during early inflammatory events are exemplified via their ability to up-regulate the expression of adherence proteins on the endothelium and allow inflammatory cells to bind to a localized area. In addition, these same cytokines can induce the expression of specific chemotactic cytokines from non-immune cells by a cascade effect known as cytokine networking. This interaction essentially transforms a bystander or target cell of the inflammatory response into an effector cell. Once the appropriate inflammatory cell has arrived at an inflammatory site, cytokines continue to be expressed and exert their influence by organizing the local immune response. Finally, the appropriate endogenous suppressive factors are expressed that initiate the resolution process. Thus, cytokines are effective transmitters of intracellular information that is crucial to each phase of an inflammatory reaction.

INTRODUCTION

Cytokines are known to comprise a group of biologically active polypeptides that are instrumental to the evolution of an inflammatory response. These polypeptide mediators are expressed by a variety of immune and non-immune cells and represent a major communication network to transmit intracellular signals during inflammation. Different cytokines are likely involved in the various facets of an inflammatory response, including the initiation, maintenance and resolution of a given reaction. Collectively, these cytokines represent polypeptide mediators with eclectic biological activities. Recent studies have demonstrated that cytokines can influence the direction of an immune response via autocrine, paracrine, and endocrine mechanisms. The ability of cytokines to exert local, regional, and systemic effects is an important concept of cytokine biology, as it addresses the pathophysiologic role of these mediators in disease. Elevation in body temperature, induction of sleep, and appetite suppression are all physiologic manifestations of disease, yet they may only represent alterations in cytokine levels that normally control circadian physiology. It is becoming increasingly clear that cytokines are involved in regulating a variety of normal physiologic events, including, diurnal body temperature, slow-wave sleep, and appetite. An increase in cytokine concentrations that are associated with inflammation may concomitantly activate inflammatory cells and alter normal physiology. Both of these events are important to the ultimate success of a host's defense response. Additional systemic effects associated with severe inflammation can also be exerted by the sustained and exaggerated production of certain cytokines. For example, patients with advanced tuberculosis may often present with multiple physiologic derangements as a potential consequence of exuberant cytokine production. In the early medical literature the disease now known as tuberculosis was called consumption, a definition that accurately reflected the physiologic state of the patient. It is now postulated that the consumption or cachexia associated with tuberculosis is due to systemic levels of tumor necrosis factor-α (TNF) or cachectin produced and released by the tubercle lesion. Fever, fatigue, and weight loss that are common symptoms of various diseases may all be mechanistically controlled by elevated levels of systemic cytokines. Thus, changes in the quantity, type, and spectrum of cytokines are key to both the pathology and physiology observed during an inflammatory response (Kunkel et al, 1989).

CYTOKINES AS MEDIATORS OF INFLAMMATION

The normal development of an inflammatory response is dependent upon cell-to-cell interactions that are mediated by a network of different signals. As described above, this group of polypeptide mediators serve important roles in establishing communication circuits that initiate, maintain, and resolve an inflammatory response. Essentially cytokines are important transmitters of information that have an important effect on a variety of target cells and are critical in regulating the host's immunologic and physiologic state (Le & Vilcek, 1987). Cytokines include an array of polypeptides, including interleukins, growth factors, and tumor necrosis factors (Table I). These factors are synthesized by an number of different cells in response to a spectrum of stimuli.

-Interleukins	-Transforming growth factor
-Colony stimulating factors	-Neutrophil chemotactic factor
-Interferons	-Monocyte chemotactic factors
-Tumor Necrosis factor-α	-Platelet derived growth factors
-Lymphotoxin	-Migration inhibitory factors

Table I. Cytokines include a number of polypeptide mediators with a multitude of biological activities. These mediators of inflammation serve as important intracellular communication circuits.

This is particularly true of the interleukin group of cytokines. The interleukin family of cytokines may represent the most well known mediators in name, but least understood in terms of function of all the cytokines. As shown in Table II, the interleukins are represented by a number of proteins derived from numerous cellular sources. Interestingly, many interleukins/cytokines possess overlapping activities, as they are important participants in the various stages of both acute and chronic inflammation (Le & Vilcek, 1987; Beutler & Cerami, 1986). This is especially evident during the initiation of either an acute or cell-mediated inflammatory response, as the proximal expression of similar cytokines appear to be important to the recruitment phase of both types of inflammation. For example, both interleukin-1 (IL-1) and tumor necrosis factor-α (TNF) appear to be key cytokines expressed early during inflammation. These polypeptide mediators are important in the induction of specific adherence proteins for both neutrophils and monocytes on the surface of endothelial cells (Pohlman et al, 1986; Schleimer et al, 1985). In addition, these proximal cytokines initiate the process necessary for the establishment of chemotactic gradients which result in the direct migration of inflammatory cells (Matsushima et al, 1988; Baggiolini et al, 1989; Westwick et al, 1989).

Interleukin	Cellular Source
IL-1α/IL-1β	Mononuclear Phagocytes/other cells
IL-2	T-Lymphocytes
IL-3	T-Lymphocytes
IL-4	T-Lymphocytes
IL-5	T-Lymphocytes
IL-6	Mononuclear Phagocytes/other cells
IL-7	T-Lymphocytes
IL-8	Mononuclear Phagocytes/other cells

Table II. Presently 8 interleukins have been identified with each possessing significant biological activity in various immune systems. Interestingly, many of the same interleukins are derived from similar cellular sources.

INFLAMMATORY CELL RECRUITMENT

The elicitation of inflammatory cells from the peripheral blood to a specific site of reactivity is a classic example of an inflammatory event mediated by a cascade of induced signals. In order for this dynamic event to occur, inflammatory cells in the lumen of a local vessel must first adhere to the endothelium, move through the endothelial cell monolayer, digest a small portion of the basement membrane, and then follow a chemotactic gradient to the site of inflammation. This entire process must be placed in perspective, as numerous physical and chemical changes are simultaneously occurring in the local vasculature (vasodilatation, leukoconcentration, and alterations in vascular permeability). Independent of this activity the inflammatory and endothelial cells must interact in a reversible manner via the expression of IL-1 and/or TNF inducible adherence proteins. This proximal event of the recruitment process has recently been addressed by a number of excellent studies, demonstrating specific surface proteins acting in a receptor-ligand manner to bind inflammatory cells to the endothelium (Pohlman et al, 1986; Schleimer & Rutledge, 1985; Springer et al, 1987). While the mechanism of adherence via CD11/CD18 expression on inflammatory cells and ICAM/ELAM expression on endothelial cells has been clarified, the more distal events of the recruitment process largely remain unknown. As shown in Table III, a variety of chemotactic factors have been identified that possess potent, but nonspecific activity. These factors have been shown to induce the directed movement of many different inflammatory cells. In addition, these chemotactic factors are relatively short lived and are susceptible to rapid degradation and clearance. Recent investigations have identified other chemotactic polypeptides which possess selective activity for neutrophils or monocytes (Table IV). Thus chemotactic cytokines appear to possess a relatively long half-life and are derived from a variety of cellular sources (Strieter et al, 1990; Elner et al, 1990; Thornton et al, 1990; Strieter et al, 1989; Strieter et al, 1989).

Chemotactic Factor	Source
Leukotriene B_4	Neutrophil/macrophages
Platelet Activating factor	Inflammatory Cells
fMLP	Bacterial metabolism
C5a	Complement activation

Table III. Chemotactic factors comprise a large collection of peptide, polypeptide, and lipid mediators. These agents are derived from a variety of sources, yet all demonstrate potent activity for moving a variety of inflammatory cells.

One of the novel peptides has been well studied and can be found in the literature under a number of different labels, including neutrophil chemotactic factor (Strieter et al, 1989), monocyte-derived neutrophil chemotactic factor (Matsushima et al, 1988), neutrophil activating peptide (Baggiolini et al, 1989), and interleukin-8 (IL-8) (Westwick et al, 1989).

Chemotactic Cytokines	Cellular Source
Interleukin-8 (IL-8)	Phagocytes/non-immune cells
GRO/MGSA	Various cells
Neutrophil activating peptide-2 (NAP2)	Platelets
Monocyte chemotactic protein (MCP)	Various cells

Table IV. Chemotactic cytokines are represented by a variety of polypeptides isolated from a number of sources. These novel mediators are important signals in mediating the recruitment of inflammatory cells.

The study of IL-8 has recently received much attention as this chemotactic cytokine is a product of many cells. In addition to mononuclear phagocytes, endothelial cells (Strieter et al, 1989), epithelial cells (Elner et al, 1990), and hepatoma cell lines (Thornton et al, 1990) have all been shown to synthesize IL-8. Although a number of cells can produce IL-8, the induction of IL-8 gene expression is stimulus specific. As shown in Table V, the mononuclear phagocytic-cells (monocytes, alveolar macrophages) can express steady state IL-8 mRNA in response to lipopolysaccharide (LPS), as well as TNF and IL-1. On the contrary, primary cultures of fibroblasts and epithelial cells are not susceptible to LPS-induced stimulation (Elner et al, 1990; Strieter et al, 1989). These noninflammatory cells appear to require an initial host response, whereby IL-1 and/or TNF is produced, prior to the generation of IL-8. The production of IL-8 by normal fibroblasts and epithelial cells by IL-1 or TNF is representative of cytokine networking. This concept is based on the ability of one cytokine to induce the expression of a second cytokine in a cascade manner.

	Adherence	LPS	Il-1	TNF	IL-6
Alveolar Macrophages	+++	++++	++++	+++	--
Blood Monocytes	++	++++	++++	+++	--
Endothelial Cells	--	+++	++++	+++	--
Fibroblasts	--	--	+++	+++	--
Hepatoma lines	--	--	+++	+++	--

Table V. Stimulus Specific Induction of IL-8 mRNA expression by immune and non-immune cells.

Our laboratory has studied cytokine networking in the lung and has demonstrated the importance of alveolar macrophage-derived IL-1 and TNF in inducing IL-8 gene expression by other non-immune lung cells. Since previous investigators from our laboratory have shown that LPS treated human alveolar macrophages are a potent source of IL-1 and TNF (Strieter et al, 1989; Strieter et al, 1989), we next tested the ability of these soluble factors to induce IL-8 from type II pneumocytes.

As shown in Figure 1, conditioned media from LPS challenged alveolar macrophages was a potent stimulus for the expression of steady state IL-8 mRNA by pulmonary type II cells. The addition of neutralizing antibodies to either IL-1β or TNF to the alveolar macrophage conditioned media significantly reduced steady state IL-8 mRNA levels by 50% and 20% respectively. These findings have a number of consequences with regard to the elicitation of inflammatory cells into the lung. A number of pulmonary diseases are characterized by the rapid recruitment of inflammatory cells into the distal airways (Hunninghake et al, 1981; McGuire et al, 1982; Hunninghake et al, 1981). Unfortunately, the mechanism(s) responsible for this chemotaxis is relatively unknown The expression of IL-8 by various cells that comprise the alveolar space/interstitium may be an important mediator for the rapid movement of cells from the pulmonary vessels into an area of lung inflammation. The importance of the alveolar macrophage as a source of cytokines in the lungs is further underscored by the ability of these cells to also secrete large levels of IL-8 (Strieter et al, 1990). Upon LPS stimulation, the alveolar macrophage can express steady state IL-8 mRNA within minutes, reach maximal expression by 8 hours, and continue to transcribe mRNA for 24 hours (Figure 2). Thus, stimulated alveolar macrophages are both a source of IL-8, produced to initiate directed movement of inflammatory cells, and a source of Il-1 and TNF, secreted to maintain the chemotactic response.

REGULATION OF TNF BY ENDOGENOUS FACTORS

The above information suggests that TNF is an important cytokine for the initiation and maintenance of an inflammatory response. A number of investigative studies have now shown that TNF is apparently under strict endogenous regulation. Both lipid and protein mediators can modulate the synthesis of TNF at the transcriptional and postranscriptional levels. Prostaglandin E_2 (PGE_2) can inhibit transcription of TNF via a cAMP-dependent mechanism (Kunkel et al, 1988; Scales et al, 1989; Spengler et al, 1989; Spengler et al, 1989). While the expression of TNF

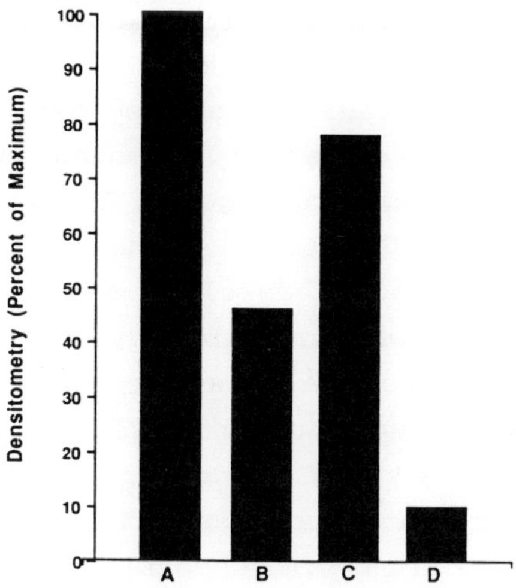

Figure 1. Laser densitometry of Northern blots demonstrating the induction of IL-8 mRNA from A549 (type II-like pneumocytes) cells treated with alveolar macrophage conditioned media, (CM). (A) LPS stimulated alveolar macrophages; (B) CM + anti-human IL-1β antibody; (C) CM + anti-human TNF antibody; and (D) CM + anti-human IL-1β and anti-TNF antibody.

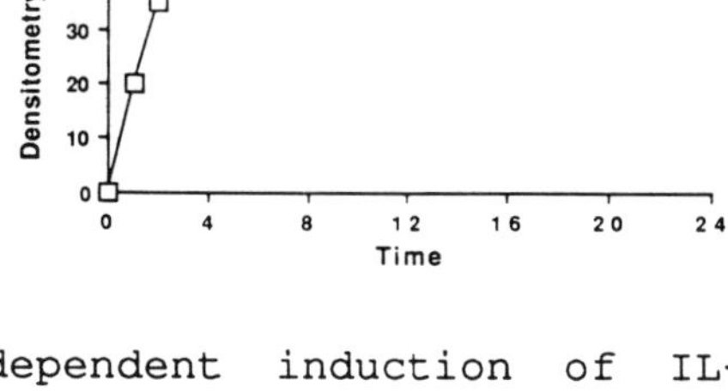

Figure 2. Time-dependent induction of IL-8 mRNA by human alveolar macrophages treated with LPS.

mRNA is rapidly induced by LPS followed by the synthesis of bioactive protein, this cytokine can be suppressed by PGE_2, forskolin, and dibutyryl cAMP in a dose-dependent manner. As shown in Table VI, each of these compounds were effective in blocking LPS-dependent macrophage TNF production. The simultaneous addition of PGE_2 (10^{-6} or 10^{-7}) plus LPS blocked the levels of TNF by about 50%. Forskolin, a compound that directly activates adenylate cyclase, and dibutyryl cAMP, a derivative of cAMP that can readily cross cellular membranes, also suppressed TNF production. These two compounds were not as effective as prostaglandins of the E series. Concentrations of dibutyryl cAMP and forskolin necessary to reduce the LPS-induced TNF response by 50% were 3×10^{-6} and 3×10^{-5}M, respectively. The time frame to modulate the production of TNF is restricted to a relatively narrow window. In an *in vitro* macrophage system, TNF synthesis is susceptible to PGE_2 or dibutyryl cAMP suppression only during a 2 to 3 hour time frame. Delaying the addition of PGE_2 for more than 2 hours after stimulating macrophages with LPS resulted in no significant suppression of TNF release.

While TNF gene expression by mononuclear phagocytic cells is regulated by PGE_2 and cAMP, the transcription and translation of an additional cytokine (IL-1) was not effected. Northern blot analysis demonstrated no effect by PGE_2 on the expression of IL-1α or IL-1-β mRNA (Scales et al, 1989). The steady state mRNA studies were further substantiated by nuclear transcription analysis of IL-1. In these studies PGE_2 did not effect the transcription of genomic IL-1 mRNA, demonstrating that PGE_2 did not block LPS induced IL-1 mRNA. Immunohistochemical experiments designed to assess antigenic cytokines further supported a disparate regulatory influence of PGE_2 on IL-1 and TNF. Immunoperioxidase staining demonstrated that PGE_2 caused a suppression of antigenic TNF but not IL-1-α or β in LPS stimulated macrophages (Scales et al, 1989). In addition, the patterns of immunolocalization were quite distinct for IL-1 and TNF, suggesting that these two cytokines were distributed differentially within the macrophage. Tumor necrosis factor appeared to be localized in specific packets in the cells, while IL-1 possessed a diffuse cytoplasmic staining pattern. This observation may have important implication as to an intracellular role for IL-1.

SUPPRESSION OF LPS-INDUCED MACROPHAGE TNF BY cAMP

	% REDUCTION		
Concentration	Dibutyryl cAMP	Forskolin	PGE_2
10^{-4}	85	90	--
10^{-5}	55	15	--
10^{-6}	30	7	60
10^{-7}	--	5	40
10^{-8}	--	--	20

Table VI. Ability of agents that increase cAMP and dibutyryl cAMP itself to inhibit TNF by LPS treated macrophages. In this study PGE_2 was more effective than forskolin or dibutyryl cAMP in regulating LPS (100 ng/ml) induced TNF production.

Additional studies have identified other polypeptide cytokines as potent mediators of IL-1 and TNF production. Both interleukin-4 (IL-4) and transforming growth factor beta (TGF-β) have been identified as suppressing LPS-dependent TNF production (Hart et al, 1989). Our laboratory has also shown that pretreatment with as little was 1.0 ng/ml of IL-4 could suppress LPS-derived TNF synthesis by activated macrophages. The concomitant addition of IL-4 also was equally as efficacious in suppressing TNF by LPS-stimulated macrophages. Especially intriguing is the ability of IL-4 to block transcription of both IL-1 and TNF. This modulation by IL-4 may represent a global macrophage suppressing cytokine, as a number of macrophage-derived mediators appear to be regulated by IL-4, including PGE_2, IL-1, TNF and GM-CSF (Hart et al, 1989). Presumably this modulation is independent of cAMP and may represent a novel intracellular signal translocation mechanism that can alter gene expression. The ability of IL-4, TGF-β, and PGE_2 to alter transcription and, in some cases, translation of TNF demonstrates the importance of the environmental "cocktail" of inflammatory mediators as being critical to the normal evolution of an immune response.

There is little doubt that both macrophages and lymphocytes are the dominant cells which possess effector and regulatory activity during cell-mediated immune reactions. Since these cells are known to exert their actions via the expression of various cytokines, it is important to understand the factors which control the production of specific cytokines.

CONCLUSION

It is becoming increasingly apparent that the field of immunology has only begun to appreciate the impact of cytokines on the inflammatory process. Attempts to clarify the exact role of these mediators during inflammation must be addressed at a multidisciplinary level. Although the contribution of molecular biologists to the cytokine field has been immeasurable, continued advances by physiologists, pharmacologists, immunologists, and pathologists will be necessary to truly understand the role of cytokines in health and disease.

ACKNOWLEDGEMENT The authors wish to thank the expert secretarial support of Suzanne Miller and Peggy Weber. This work was supported in part by NIH grants HL31693, HL35276, and DK38149. Steven L. Kunkel is an established investigator of the American Heart Association.

REFERENCES

Baggiolini, M., Walz, A., and Kunkel, S.L. (1989) NAP-/IL-8, a novel cytokine that activates neutrophils. J. Clin. Invest 84;1045-1049.

Beutler, B. and Cerami, A. (1986) Cachectin and tumor necrosis factor as two sides of the same biological coin. Nature, 320:584-588.

Elner, V.M., Strieter, R.M., Elner, S.G., Baggiolini, M., Lindley, I, and Kunkel, S.L. (1990) Neutrophil chemo- tactic factor (IL-8) gene expression by cytokine treated retinal pigment epithelial cells. Am. J. Pathol. 136:745-750.

Hart, P.H., Vitti, G.F., Burgess, D.R., Whitty, G.A., Piccoli, D.S., and Hamilton, J.A. (1989) Potential anti-inflammatory effects of interleukin-4: Suppression of human monocyte tumor necrosis factor-α, interleukin-1, and prostaglandin E_2. Proc. Natl. Acad. Sci. USA 86:3803-3807.

Hunninghake, G.W., Kawanami, O., Ferrans, V.J., Roberts, W.C., and Crystal, R.G. (1981) Characterization of the inflammatory and immune effector cells in the lung parenchyma of patients with interstitial lung disease. Am. Rev. Respir. Dis. 123:407-418.

Hunninghake, G.W., Gadek, J.E., Lawley, T.J., and Crystal, R.G. (1981) Mechanisms of neutrophil accumulation in the lungs of patients with idiopathic pulmonary fibrosis. J. Clin. Invest. 68:259-267.

Kunkel, S.L., Chensue, S.W., Strieter, R.M, Lynch, J.P., and Remick D.G. (1989) Cellular and molecular aspects of granuloma formation. Am. J. Respir. Cell. Mol. Biol. 1:439-447.

Kunkel, S.L., Spengler, M., May, M.A., Spengler, R., Larrick, J. and Remick, D.G. (1988) Prostaglandin E_2 regulates macrophage-derived tumor necrosis factor gene expression. J. Biol. Chem. 263:5380-5384.

Le, J. and Vilcek, J. (1987) Tumor necrosis factor and interleukin-1: Cytokines with multiple overlapping biological activities. Lab. Invest. 56:234-245.

Matsushima, K., Morishita, K., Yoshimura, T., Lavu, S., Kobayashi, Y., Lew, W., Apella, E., Kung, H.F., Leonard, E. J., and Oppenheim, J.J. (1988) Molecular cloning of a human monocyte-derived neutrophil chemotactic factor (MDNCF) and the induction of MDNCF mRNA by interleukin-1 and tumor necrosis factor. J. Exp. Med. 167:1883-1893.

McGuire, W.W., Spragg, R.G., Cohen, A.B., and Cochran, C.G. (1982) Studies on the pathogenesis of the adult respiratory distress syndrome. J. Clin. Invest. 69:543-555.

Pohlman, T.H., Stanness, K.A., Beatty, P.G., Ochs, H.D., and Harlan, J.M. (1986) An endothelial cell surface factor(s) induced *in vitro* by lipopolysaccharide, interleukin-1, and tumor necrosis factor alpha increase neutrophil adherence by a CDW 18-dependent mechanism. J. Immunol. 136:4548-4559.

Scales, W.E., Chensue, S.W., Otterness, I., and Kunkel, S.L. Regulation of monokine gene expression: Prostaglandin E suppresses TNF but not IL-1α or β mRNA and cell associated bioactivity. J. Leuko. Biol. 45:416-421.

Schleimer, R.P. and Rutledge, B.K. (1985) Cultured human vascular endothelium acquires adhesiveness for neutrophils after stimulation with interleukin-1, endotoxin, and tumor promoting phorbol diesters. J. Immunol. 136:649-660.

Spengler, R.N., Spengler, M.L., Lincoln, P., Remick, D.G., Strieter, R.M., and Kunkel, S.L. (1989) Dynamics of dibutyryl cAMP and prostaglandin E-mediated suppression of lipopolysaccharide induced tumor necrosis factor alpha gene expression. Infect. Immun. 57:2837-2841.

Spengler, R.N., Spengler, M.L, Strieter, R.M., Remick, D.G., Larrick J.W., and Kunkel, S.L. (1989) Modulation of tumor necrosis factor alpha gene expression: Desensitization of prostaglandin E-induced suppression. J. Immunol. 142:4346-4350.

Springer, T.A., Dustin, M.L., Kishimoto, T.K, and Marlin, S.D. (1987) The lymphocyte function-associated LFA-1, cD2, and LFA_3 molecules: Cell adhesions receptor of the immune system. Annu. Rev. Immunol. 5:223-252.

Strieter, R.M., Chensue, S.W., Basha, M.A., Standiford, T.J., Lynch, J.P. III, Baggiolini, M., and Kunkel, S.L. (1990) Human alveolar macrophage gene expression of interleukin-8 by tumor necrosis factor-α, lipopoly- saccharide, and interleukin-1β. Am. J. Respir. Cell Moll. Biol. 2:321-326.

Strieter, R.M., Remick, D.G., Lynch, J.P. III, Spengler, R.N., and Kunkel, S.L. (1989) Interleukin-2 induced tumor necrosis factor-α (TNF) gene expression in human alveolar macrophages and blood monocytes. Am. Rev. Respir. Dis. 139:335-342.

Strieter, R.M., Remick, D.G., Lynch, J.P. III, and Kunkel, S.L. (1989) Differential regulation of tumor necrosis factor in human alveolar macrophages and peripheral blood monocytes: A cellular and molecular analysis. Am. J. Respir. Cell. Mol. Biol. 1:57-63.

Strieter, R.M., Kunkel, S.L., Showell, H.J., Remick, D.G., Phan, S.H., Ward, P.A., and Marks, R.M. (1989) Monokine-induced neutrophil chemotactic factor gene expression in human fibroblasts. J. Biol. Chem. 264:10621-10626.

Strieter, R.M., Kunkel, S.L., Showell, H.J., Remick, D.G., Phan, S.H., Ward, P.A., and Marks, R.M. (1989) Endothelial cell gene expression a neutrophil chemotactic factor by TNF-α, LPS, and IL-1β. Science 243:1467-1469.

Thornton, A.J., Strieter, R.M., Lindley, I., Baggiolini, M., and Kunkel, S.L. (1990) Cytokine-induced gene expres- sion of a neutrophil chemotactic factor/IL-8 in human hepatocytes. J. Immunol. 144:2609-2613.

Westwick, J., Li, S.W., and Camp, R.D. (1989) Purification of a human monocyte-derived neutrophil-derived chemo- tactic factor that shares sequence homology with other host defense cytokines. Immunol. Today 10:146-148.

P52390.slk/csm

AAS 32
Drugs in Inflammation

ANTIINFLAMMATORY PROPERTIES OF E5090, A NOVEL ORALLY ACTIVE INHIBITOR OF IL-1 GENERATION

H. Shirota, K. Chiba, M. Goto, R. Hashida and H. Ono

Eisai Tsukuba Research Laboratories, 5-1-3 Tokodai, Tsukuba, Ibaraki 300-26, Japan

SUMMARY: E5090 is a novel orally active inhibitor of IL-1 generation without cyclooxygenase-inhibiting activity. The effects of E5090 on several inflammatory animal models were investigated in rats. In adjuvant arthritis, E5090 suppressed both the paw swelling and the enhancements of ESR and number of peripheral blood leucocytes, like the steroidal antiinflammatory drug prednisolone. However, the thymus was not withered by E5090 though it was by prednisolone. In type II collagen-induced arthritis, E5090 inhibited paw swelling and joint destruction. E5090 was effective in acute inflammatory models such as carrageenin-induced paw edema, and adjuvant-induced local hyperthermia, and also showed analgesic effects against inflammatory pain and antipyretic effects. The results suggest that this orally active inhibitor of IL-1 generation, E5090, may be a therapeutically useful antiinflammatory drug with a novel mechanism of action.

INTRODUCTION

Many reports concerning interleukin-1 (IL-1) have indicated that IL-1 plays important roles in inflammation. E5090, (Z)-3-[4-(acetyloxy)-5-ethyl-3-methoxy-1-naphthalenyl]-2-methyl-2-propenoic acid, is a newly synthesized orally active inhibitor of IL-1 generation[1,2] without cyclooxygenase-inhibiting activity. The present study was conducted to clarify the antiinflammatory properties of E5090 using various acute and chronic inflammatory animal models.

MATERIALS AND METHODS

Drugs: E5090 was synthesized in our laboratories. As reference drugs, prednisolone (PRED, Wako Junyaku Co.) and indomethacin (IND, Sigma Chemical Co.) were used. These drugs were suspended in 0.5% methylcellulose solution and administered orally in the following experiments.

Effects on chronic inflammatory models: Adjuvant arthritis was provoked by the injection of *M. butyricum* into the right hind paw of male Fisher (F344) rats. The test drugs were orally administered once daily from the 1st day to the 17th day after the adjuvant injection. Changes in swelling of both adjuvant-treated and -untreated paws were determined. The erythrocyte sedimentation rate (ESR), peripheral blood leucocyte number (PBL), serum α1-acid glycoprotein (AGP), and the weights of immunologically significant organs were measured on the 18th day after the adjuvant injection.

Type II collagen-induced arthritis was prepared by immunization with bovine type II collagen at the dorsal site of male Lewis rats. The test drugs were orally administered from the 1st day to the 27th day after the immunization. Changes in paw swelling were determined, and the degrees of joint destruction were also determined by X-ray radiography on the 28th day after the immunization.

Effects on acute inflammatory models: The effects of E5090 on carrageenin-induced paw edema[3)] and adjuvant-induced local hyperthermia[4)] were examined in male SD and Fisher rats, respectively. The Arthus pleurisy[5)] was used as an allergic inflammatory model. In this model, IL-1 and PGE2 contents in the exudates were measured by standard LAF assay and RIA, respectively.

Analgesic effects: To determine the analgesic effects of E5090 against inflammatory pain, both the lame walking reaction test[5)] in rats with acute paw inflammation and the flection pain test[5)] in rats with chronic adjuvant arthritis were employed.

Antipyretic effects: To determine the antipyretic effects of E5090 on febrile rats, both lipopolysaccharide (LPS)-induced pyrexia, which was provoked by the i.v. injection of 10μg/kg of LPS, and baker's yeast-induced pyrexia[5] were used.

RESULTS AND DISCUSSION

Table I. Values of minimum effective dose (mg/kg, p.o.) of E5090 and the reference drugs in some inflammatory animal models.

Animal models		E5090	PRED	IND
Chronic inflammatory models				
Adjuvant-arthritis	paw sweling	25	2.5	≦1
	ESR	100	10	NE
	No. of PBL	50	10	NE
	α1-AGP	100-200	5-10	NE
	thymus atrophy	NE	1.25 (AV)	1
	splenomegaly	100	2.5	NE
Collagen-arthritis	paw swelling	25	2.5	≦1
	joint destruction	25	2.5	≦1
Acute inflammatory models				
Carrageenin-paw edema		100	5	1
Adjuvant-local hyperthermia		10-30	1	0.3
Arthus pleurisy	Exudate volume	10	NT	NT
	PGE2 content	>100	NT	NT
	IL-1 content	30	NT	NT
Inflammatory pain				
Lame walking reaction		50	5	≦3
Arthritic flection pain		25	5	1
Pyrexia				
LPS-induced pyrexia		50	10	2.5-10
Yeast-induced pyrexia		10-30	1-3	≦3

NT means not tested. NE means not effective. AV means aggravation.

Table I shows the effects of E5090 and the reference drugs on various inflammatory animal models. In adjuvant arthritis, E5090 suppressed not only paw inflammation but also the enhancements of ESR, PBL number, and α1-AGP, being similar to PRED in these respects, but different from IND. In this arthritic model, the thymus weights were decreased and the spleen weights were increased as compared with normal rats. Both E5090 and PRED improved the splenomegaly. On the other hand, E5090 had no effect on the thymus atrophy, while PRED aggravated it. These results suggest that the efficacy of E5090 in this model is similar to that of steroids, but E5090 does not exhibit steroid-like immunological toxicities. In type II collagen arthritis, E5090 suppressed both paw swelling and joint destruction. The inhibition of prostaglandins may be more effective in this arthritic model because the treatment with IND caused more significant suppression than that with E5090. However, it is of great importance that this inhibitor of IL-1 generation without cyclooxygenase-inhibiting activity, E5090, exhibits an improvement of joint destruction in this model. The inhibitory potency of E5090 in these arthritic models was estimated to be about 1/10 of that of PRED.

In addition, E5090 was effective in acute inflammatory models such as carrageenin-induced paw edema and adjuvant-induced local hyperthermia, and also showed analgesic effects against inflammatory pain and antipyretic effects. It is accepted that these acute inflammatory models are very sensitive to inhibitors of prostaglandins generation but insensitive to some disease-modifying antirheumatic drugs such as aurotiomalate, D-penicillamine, lobenzarit and so on. An orally active inhibitor of IL-1 generation, E5090, showed antiinflammatory effects in all these models, indicating that IL-1 also has important roles in these acute inflammation models.

In conclusion, E5090 appears to be an antiinflammatory drug with a novel mechanism of action, and it may be especially useful in the treatment of rheumatoid arthritis.

REFERENCES

1) Goto, M., Chiba, K., Hashida, R. and Shirota, H. (1990) A novel inhibitor of IL-1 generation, E5090: In vitro effects on the generation of IL-1 by human monocytes, Agents and Actions, accompanying paper.
2) Chiba, K., Goto, M. and Shirota, H. (1990) A novel inhibitor of IL-1 generation, E5090: In vivo inhibitory effect on the generation of IL-1-like factor and on granuloma formation in an air-pouch model, Agents and Actions, accompanying paper.
3) Winter, C.A., Risley, E.A. and Nuss, G.W. (1962) Carrageenin-induced edema in hind paw of the rat as an assay for anti-inflammatory drugs., Proc. Soc. Exp. Biol. Med. 111, 544-547.
4) Shirota, H., Goto, M. and Katayama, K. (1988) Application of adjuvant-induced local hyperthermia for evaluation of anti-inflammatory drugs., J. Pharmacol. Exp. Ther. 247, 1158-1163.
5) Shirota, H., Chiba, K., Ono, H., Yamamoto, H., Kobayashi, S., Terato, K., Ikuta, H., Yamatsu, I. and Katayama, K. (1987) Pharmacological properties of novel non-steroidal anti-inflammatory agent N-methoxy-3-(3,5-di-tert-butyl-4-hydroxybenzylidene)pyrrolidin-2-one., Arzneim.-Forsch./ Drug Res. 37, 930-936.

AAS 32
Drugs in Inflammation

A NOVEL INHIBITOR OF IL-1 GENERATION, E5090: *IN VITRO* INHIBITORY EFFECTS ON THE GENERATION OF IL-1 BY HUMAN MONOCYTES

M. Goto, K. Chiba, R. Hashida and H. Shirota

Eisai Research Laboratories, Eisai Co., Ltd., 5-1-3 Tokodai, Tsukuba, Ibaraki 300-26, Japan

SUMMARY: E5090 is an orally active inhibitor of IL-1 generation, being converted *in vivo* into the pharmacologically active deacetylated form (DA-E5090). *In vitro* effects of DA-E5090 on the generation of IL-1 by human monocytes stimulated with LPS were examined. DA-E5090 inhibited both IL-1α and IL-1β generation by human monocytes stimulated with 1 μg/ml of LPS in a dose dependent-manner (1-10 μM), as determined by LAF assay and ELISA. Northern blotting analysis indicated that DA-E5090 inhibits transcription of IL-1α and IL-1β m-RNAs.

INTRODUCTION

Interleukin-1 (IL-1) is a cytokine with various biological actions, and is mainly produced by stimulated macrophages/monocytes. Recent studies have suggested that IL-1 may play important roles in rheumatoid arthritis (RA) because of its stimulation of synovial cells to release PGE_2 and collagenase, its activation of hepatocytes to synthesize and release acute-phase proteins and its action on chondrocytes to cause cartilage degradation (Dinarello, C.A., 1989). Therefore, it is rational to consider that an inhibitor of IL-1 generation could be a useful therapeutic agent in the treatment of RA.

E5090, (Z)-3-[4-(acetyloxy)-5-ethyl-3-methoxy-1-naphthalenyl]-2-

methyl-2-propenoic acid, is a newly synthesized and orally active inhibitor of IL-1 generation (Chiba, K, et al.,1990). Orally administered E5090 is rapidly absorbed and transformed to the deacetylated form (DA-E5090), which is the pharmacologically active form. This paper describes the inhibitory effects of DA-E5090 on the generation of IL-1 by human monocytes.

MATERIALS AND METHODS

IL-1 generation by human monocytes: Human monocytes from peripheral blood of healthy volunteers were obtained by the method previously reported (Oppenheim,J.J. et al., 1976). The cells were suspended in RPMI 1640 containing 10% heat-inactivated autologous serum, seeded into 48-well plastic culture plates (1-2 x 10^6 cells/0.5 ml), and cultured at 37°C for 1.5 hours. Non adherent cells were removed by rinsing, and the remaining cells were used as the monocyte preparation. The monocytes were cultured with 1 µg/ml of lipopolysaccharide (LPS from *E. coli* serotype 0127:B8) in the presence or absence of DA-E5090 at 37°C for 16-18 hours. The medium was RPMI 1640 with 1% heat-inactivated autologous serum, 0.1% ethanol, 100 units/ml of penicillin, and 100 µg/ml of streptomycin. Then, the culture supernatant was collected, and filtered with a Millipore filter (0.22 µm), and the IL-1 content in the filtrate was determined. To measure intracellular IL-1, 0.5 ml of RPMI 1640 was added to the well after removal of the supernatant, and the cells were homogenized by sonication.

Determination of IL-1: IL-1 activity was determined by the standard LAF assay (Oppenheim, J.J. et al., 1976). The amounts of IL-1 in the test samples, which were serially diluted, were calculated from a titration curve prepared with standard human recombinant IL-1β (Genzyme). Amounts of IL-1 proteins were determined by using IL-1α and IL-1β ELISA kits (Otsuka Pharmaceutical Co., Ltd.).

Northern blotting analysis of IL-1 m-RNA expression.: Human monocytes were cultured for 4 hours with 1 μg/ml of LPS in RPMI 1640 containing 1% autologous serum in the presence or absence of DA-E5090. RNA isolation and northern blotting analysis were carried out as described (Sambrook, J. et al., 1989) by using DNA probes of human IL-1α, IL-1β and β-actin.

RESULTS

Inhibitory Effect of DA-E5090 on the generation of IL-1 by human monocytes stimulated with LPS: When human monocytes were stimulated with LPS (1 μg/ml) for 18 hours, IL-1 activities were detected in both culture supernatant and cells. DA-E5090 reduced IL-1 activity, determined by LAF assay, in a dose-dependent manner (Table I). The inhibitory effects of DA-E5090 were also investigated by ELISA of IL-1α and IL-1β. IL-1α mainly existed within the cells, while IL-1β existed in the culture supernatant. DA-E5090 reduced the amounts of both IL-1α and IL-1β.

Inhibitory effect of DA-E5090 on expression of IL-1 m-RNA in human monocytes: In order to examine whether the inhibitory effect of DA-E5090 on IL-1 generation is caused by suppression of IL-1 m-RNA expression, northern blotting analysis was performed. DA-E5090 reduced the expression of both IL-1α m-RNA and IL-1β m-RNA (Fig. 1). The levels of β-actin m-RNA were unchanged by treatment with DA-E5090.

DISCUSSION

E5090 is an orally active inhibitor of IL-1 generation in rat air-pouch models (Chiba, K. et al., 1990), and it exhibits anti-inflammatory effects in various inflammatory animal models (Shirota, H. et al., 1990). E5090 itself has little or no inhibitory effect on IL-1 generation, but orally administered E5090 is

Table I. INHIBITORY EFFECT OF DA-E5090 ON IL-1 GENERATION BY HUMAN MONOCYTES STIMULATED WITH LPS

	LAF (units/ml)		ELISA (pg/ml)			
			IL-1α		IL-1β	
	sup	cell	sup	cell	sup	cell
medium	4.4	4.2	0	0	0	0
LPS	46.2	44.0	106	1286	1114	241
+DA-E5090 1μM	49.0	27.4	72	792	929	147
3	27.4	29.9	61	620	748	49
10	13.0	7.1	52	175	377	33

Each value is the mean of triplicate samples.

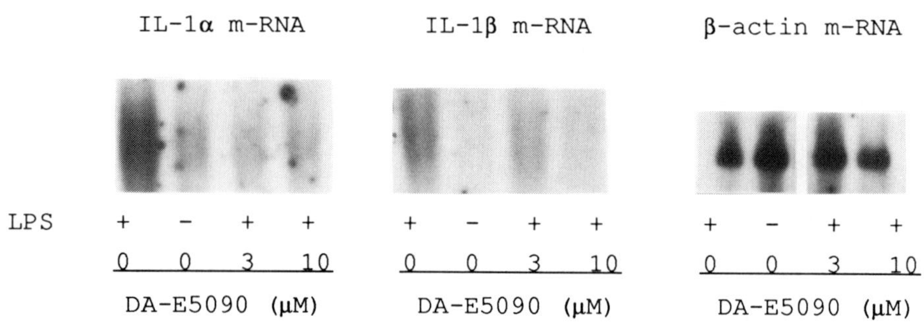

Fig.1 EFFECT OF DA-E5090 ON EXPRESSION OF IL-1α, IL-1β and β-actin m-RNAs

Cellular RNA of human monocytes was extracted and analyzed by northern blot hybridization using radiolabeled DNA probe of human IL-1α, IL-1β and β-actin.

rapidly absorbed and transformed to the pharmacologically active DA-E5090, which circulates in peripheral blood. The results presented here demonstrate that DA-E5090 inhibits both IL-1α and IL-1β generation by human monocytes based on the inhibition of IL-1 m-RNA expression. DA-E5090 had no inhibitory effect on either [^{35}S]methionine incorporation (data not shown) or β-actin m-RNA expression. These results suggest the inhibitory effect of DA-E5090 on IL-1 generation is not due to non-specific inhibition of protein or m-RNA biosynthesis.

The inhibitory effects of DA-E5090 on IL-1 generation are commonly observed in several _in vitro_ systems using not only human monocytes but also rat and mouse exudate macrophages activated with various stimuli such as LPS, opsonized zymosan and immune complexes, and thus are similar to those of the steroidal antiinflammatory drug, prednisolone (data not shown). These findings suggest that E5090 may be useful in the treatment of some inflammatory diseases, especially RA.

In conclusion, DA-E5090, the pharmacologically active form of E5090, inhibits IL-1 generation at the step of transcription of IL-1 m-RNA in human monocytes.

REFERENCES

Chiba,K., Goto,M. and Shirota,H. (1990) A novel inhibitor of IL-1 generation, E5090; In vivo inhibitory effects on the generation of IL-1 like factor and on granuloma formation in air-pouch model. Agents and Actions, accompanying paper.

Dinarello,C.A. (1989) Interleukin-1 and Its Biologically Related Cytokines. Advances In Immunology 44, 153-205.

Oppenheim,J.J., Shneyour,A. and Kook,A.I. (1976) Enhancement of DNA Synthesis and cAMP content of mouse thymocytes by mediator(s) derived from adherent cells, J.Immunol. 116, 1466-1472.

Sambrook,J., Fritsch,E.F. and Maniatis,T. (1989) Extraction, Purification, and Analysis of Messenger RNA from Eukariotic Cells. Molecular Cloning, 2nd ed., vol.1, chapter 7.Cold Spring Harbor Labolatory Press, New York.

Shirota,H., Chiba,K., Goto,M., Hashida,R. and Ono,H.(1990) Anti-inflammatory properties of E5090, A novel orally active inhibitor of IL-1 generation. Agents and Actions, accompanying paper.

AAS 32
Drugs in Inflammation

A NOVEL INHIBITOR OF IL-1 GENERATION, E5090: *IN VIVO* INHIBITORY EFFECT ON THE GENERATION OF IL-1-LIKE FACTOR AND ON GRANULOMA FORMATION IN AN AIR-POUCH MODEL.

K. Chiba, M. Goto and H. Shirota

Eisai Tsukuba Research Laboratories, 5-1-3 Tokodai, Tsukuba, Ibaraki 300-26, Japan

SUMMARY: The *in vivo* production of IL-1-like activity was investigated in the exudate of a rat air-pouch inflammatory model. An inflammatory reaction was induced by LPS injection into the air-pouch. IL-1 activity in the exudate reached the maximum level at 4 h and then rapidly decreased until 8 h after the injection of LPS. Orally administered E5090 and prednisolone dose-dependently inhibited the generation of IL-1 activity. Both compounds also suppressed chronic granuloma formation in parallel with the IL-1 inhibition. On the other hand, indomethacin had no effect on either IL-1 generation or granuloma formation in spite of the complete inhibition of PGE_2 generation. These results suggest that E5090 inhibits the production of IL-1-like activity in the exudate and exhibits steroid-like antiinflammatory effects.

INTRODUCTION

Orally administered E5090 is rapidly absorbed and immediately transformed to the pharmacologically active form (DA-E5090) by deacetylation. As shown in the preceding paper, DA-E5090 is a potent inhibitor of interleukin-1 (IL-1) generation.

IL-1 is a polypeptide and has multiple biological activities.

For example, it induces the production of prostaglandins and collagenase from synovial cells. Fibroblast proliferation and collagen biosynthesis are also stimulated by IL-1. Based on these *in vitro* activities, IL-1 is thought to play important roles in chronic inflammation.

Rheumatoid arthritis (RA) is a representative chronic inflammatory disease and the importance of IL-1 in RA has been reported by various investigators. Therefore, an *in vivo* inflammatory model suitable to allow quantitative measurements of IL-1 in the inflammatory foci is necessary to help in the search for novel anti-inflammatory and/or anti-rheumatic drugs.

In this paper, we describe a rat air-pouch inflammation model in which IL-1-like activity in the inflammatory exudate can be determined. The effects of E5090 on this model were investigated.

MATERIALS AND METHODS

Animals: Male 6-week-old Fisher strain (F_{344}) rats were obtained from Charles River Japan.

Drugs: E5090, (Z)-3-[4-(acetyloxy)-5-ethyl-3-methoxy-1-naphthalenyl]-2-methyl-2-propenoic acid, was synthesized in our laboratories. Prednisolone (PRED) was purchased from Wako Pure Chemical Ind. and indomethacin (IND) was from Sigma Chemicals.

Induction of CMC-LPS air-pouch inflammation model: A volume of 10 ml of air was injected subcutaneously at the dorsum of rats. At 24 h after the injection of air, 6 ml of a sterilized 2% (w/v) sodium carboxymethyl cellulose (CMC-Na, Cellogen F-3H, Dai-ichikogyo Seiyaku Co.) in saline was injected into the air-pouch. Inflammation was induced by injecting 5 ng of lipopolysaccharide (LPS, Sigma) dissolved in 0.5 ml of saline 24 h after the CMC injection.

Effects of E5090, and steroidal and non-steroidal antiinflammato-

ry drugs: E5090, PRED and IND were administered orally 2 h before the LPS injection. At 4 h after the LPS injection, 50 μl of inflammatory exudate was collected from the air-pouch for measurements of IL-1 activity and PGE_2 content. As inflammatory signs, serum concentration of α_1-acid glycoprotein (AGP) and granuloma wet weight were determined at 24 h and 5 days after the LPS injection, respectively.

Measurement of IL-1-like activity in the exudate: The exudate samples were diluted with 5% heat-inactivated FCS-RPMI 1640 medium and centrifuged. The cell-free supernatants containing the extracellular IL-1 were stored at -80°C until assay. The pellets were resuspended in the same medium and homogenized by sonication for measurements of intracellular IL-1, and the homogenates were stored at -80°C. The extra- and intracellular IL-1 activities were measured by a thymocyte proliferation assay (Oppenheim et al., 1976). The amount of IL-1 was calculated by using a standard curve prepared with human recombinant IL-1α (Genzyme). The total amount of IL-1 in the exudate was calculated by the summation of extra- and intracellular IL-1 contents.

PGE_2 determination: The amount of PGE_2 in the exudate supernatant was determined by using a radioimmunoassay kit (New England Nuclear).

AGP determination: The serum concentration of AGP was determined by the quantitative precipitin technique (Jamieson et al., 1972).

RESULTS AND DISCUSSION

The sequential injections of CMC and LPS into the one-day air-pouch induced inflammation accompanied with increases in IL-1-like activity and PGE_2. IL-1 activity in the exudate was mainly detected intracellularly. Total IL-1 activity reached a maximum 4 h after the LPS injection and then rapidly decreased until 8 h. PGE_2 was detected only in the supernatant and showed a similar time-course to IL-1 activity.

The effects of E5090, and steroidal and non-steroidal anti-inflammatory drugs on the CMC-LPS air-pouch model were examined. As shown in Table I, orally administered E5090 dose-dependently inhibited the generations of IL-1 activity and PGE_2, similarly to PRED. The inhibitory potency of E5090 on IL-1 generation was estimated to be about 1/10 of that of PRED. E5090 and PRED also suppressed the acute phase (serum AGP level) and the chronic

Table I.
Effects of E5090, and steroidal and non-steroidal antiinflammatory drugs on IL-1 and PGE_2 at 4 h, AGP at 24 h, and granuloma at 5 days in the CMC-LPS air-pouch model.

DRUG	DOSE (mg/kg)	IL-1 (U/ml)	PGE_2 (ng/ml)	AGP (mg/ml)	GRANULOMA WET WEIGHT (g)
[Experiment 1]					
Control		3343.2±704.8	43.5±8.3	1.40±0.07	2.079±0.109
E5090	25	2226.7±469.0	15.4±3.1*	1.34±0.10	1.964±0.059
	50	1244.9±160.7*	7.8±1.8*	0.95±0.11*	1.662±0.051*
	100	800.7±189.8*	3.0±0.5*	0.82±0.07*	1.473±0.124*
	200	331.6±16.9*	2.1±0.4*	0.91±0.11*	1.240±0.080*
PRED	5	1006.0±122.6*	11.6±1.7*	1.34±0.05	1.758±0.136
	10	661.4±77.3*	10.0±1.6*	1.08±0.12*	1.655±0.081*
	20	527.5±26.1*	6.7±1.5*	0.95±0.10*	1.416±0.046*
LPS(-)		N.D.	N.D.	0.59±0.04*	1.170±0.013*
[Experiment 2]					
Control		3766.0±397.1	24.1±4.8	1.16±0.07	2.590±0.135
E5090	100	360.6±61.2*	0.5±0.3*	0.83±0.12	1.554±0.144*
IND	3	3632.1±661.7	0.7±0.5*	1.06±0.11	2.420±0.168
LPS(-)		N.D.	N.D.	0.31±0.22*	1.237±0.120*

* $p<0.05$ vs Control. N.D. means not detected.

phase (granuloma formation) responses by single administration at 2 h before the LPS injection. On the other hand, IND had no effect on IL-1 generation or on these inflammatory signs, in spite of the complete inhibition of PGE_2 generation.

AGP is one of the acute-phase proteins induced by cytokines, especially IL-1, in rats (Andus et al., 1988). The participation of IL-1 in granuloma formation has been demonstrated (Kasahara et al., 1988), and therefore, the steroid-like antiinflammatory effects of E5090 may be caused by the suppression of IL-1 production in the acute phase of inflammation. In fact, when E5090 was administered at 24 h after the LPS injection, no inhibitory effect on granuloma formation was seen (data not shown).

In conclusion, by using this model, it was clearly demonstrated that orally administered E5090 inhibited the generation of IL-1-like factor in the inflammatory exudate. Further, it was found that E5090 exhibited steroid-like antiinflammatory effects, probably through its inhibition of IL-1 production.

REFERENCES

Andus,T., Geiger, T., Hirano, T., Kishimoto, T. and Heinrich, P.C.(1988) Action of recombinant human interleukin 6, interleukin 1β and tumor necrosis factor α on the mRNA induction of acute-phase proteins. Eur J Immunol 18,739-746.

Jamieson, J.C., Ashton. F.E., Friesen,A.D. and Chou, B. (1972) Studies on acute phase proteins of rat serum. II. Determination of the contents of α_1-acid glycoprotein, α_2-macroglobulin, and albumin in serum from rats suffering from induced inflammation. Can J Biochem 50, 871-880.

Kasahara, K., Kobayashi, K., Shikama, Y., Yoneya, I., Soezima,K., Ide, H. and Takahashi, T. (1988) Direct evidence for granuloma-inducing activity of interleukin-1. Induction of experimental pulmonary granuloma formation in mice by interleukin-1-coupled beads. Am J Pathol 130, 629-638.

Oppenheim, J.J., Shneyour, A. and Kook, A.I.(1976) Enhancement of DNA synthesis and cAMP content of mouse thymocytes by mediator(s) derived from adherent cells. J Immunol 116, 1466-1472.

AAS 32
Drugs in Inflammation

LACK OF ADJUVANTICITY OF HUMAN RECOMBINANT INTERLEUKIN-1β IN COLLAGEN INDUCED ARTHRITIS IN RATS.

P. Fener[1], P. Gillet[1], G. Charrière[2], B. Bannwarth[1], E. Drelon[1], J.Y. Jouzeau[1], D. Chevrier[1], B. Terlain[3], J. Pourel[1], D.J. Hartmann[2], P. Netter[1]

1. Laboratoire de Pharmacologie et Clinique Rhumatologique, URA CNRS 1288, Faculté de Médecine, F 54505 VANDOEUVRE-LES-NANCY
2. Centre de Radio-Analyse, Institut Pasteur, URA CNRS 602, F 69366 LYON
3. Rhône-Poulenc Santé, F 94400 VITRY SUR SEINE, FRANCE.

SUMMARY: We investigated the influence of human recombinant interleukin-1β (hrIL-1β) on the time-course of collagen induced arthritis (CIA) when injected concomitantly with the arthritogenic emulsion. Three sensitizing procedures were compared. The control group received type II collagen only. The other groups differed by the adjunction of demonstrated (MDP) or potential (IL-1β) adjuvant. No adjuvant effect of IL-1 was observed as judged on clinical or radiological scores. On the contrary, MDP significantly worsened the lesions of the injected right hindpaw, and increased the incidence of CIA. Surprisingly, humoral response to type II collagen was decreased in the group receiving IL-1β. This might be explained by a non specific increase of antigen clearance.

Interleukin-1 (IL-1) plays a central role in various inflammatory processes including rheumatoid arthritis. It acts in vitro as an amplifier of the inflammatory reaction, and may enhance, in vivo, the secondary antibody responses to a protein antigen in mice (Staruch and Wood, 1983).

It was reported that muramyl dipeptide (MDP), when added to the antigen emulsion (type II collagen (CII) + Freund's incomplete adjuvant (FIA)), increases the incidence of collagen induced arthritis (CIA) in rats (Koga et al, 1980). This adjuvant effect of MDP was attributed to the release of IL-1 from macrophages (Vacheron et al, 1983). We investigated, therefore, the influence of MDP and of human recombinant interleukin-1β (hrIL-1β) on the course of CIA in rats.

MATERIALS AND METHODS

Thirty-six female inbred Wistar-Furth rats, weighting 170-195 g, were divided in 3 batches of 12 rats as follows:

- group A (control group): rats were immunized with 80 µg of human native CII (hnCII) (Bioetica, Lyon, France) solubilized in 0.3 ml acetic acid 0.5 M, and emulsified with 0.3 ml FIA (Difco Laboratory, Detroit, USA). On day 0, the emulsion was injected subcutaneously into the rear right hindpaw (0.3 ml) and the base of the tail (0.5ml). A booster injection (15 µg hnCII +FIA) was given on day 14 into the base of the tail.
- group B (MDP group): MDP (200 µg) (Choay Réactifs Chimie, France) was added to the collagen emulsion. Muramyl dipeptide could be arthritogenic by itself, but a higher dosage is usually required (Gillet et al, 1989).
- group C (IL-1 group): hrIL-1β (0.2 mg) was added to the antigen emulsion. The dose of 0.2 µg of hrIL-1β had been chosen in accordance with the literature data (Jacobs et al, 1988) and with a previous personal unpublished dose-ranging study. HrIL-1β was provided by Rhône Poulenc Santé.

Arthritis assessment:

.Clinical scores : A score graded 0 to 4 was allocated to each of the 3 non-injected paws. The systemic disease was evaluated with an arthritic index summed from scores of the 3 non-injected paws (maximum score: 12 per rat) (Fener et al, 1990). In addition, soft tissue inflammation of the injected hindpaw was assessed with a similar scale graded 0-4.

.Plethysmography : The volume of the two hindpaws was measured up to the skin-coat partition of the hindpaw using a mercury plethysmograph (ΔV 3 model, UGO BASILE, MILAN).

Clinical scores, weight (electronic scale) and hindpaw volume were regularly determined until sacrifice (day 32).

.X Ray examination: after euthanasia (day 32), the left hindpaws were collected. Radiographs were performed using an X-Ray tube (CGR) with a microfocal spot 0.6, and using KODAK fine screens with single emulsion 18x24 cm. Joint lesions and periosteal new bone formation were each blindly graded 0-6 as previously described (Fener et al, 1990).

.Immunoassay of antibodies to collagen: Sera were collected on day 32 by cardiac puncture. Antibodies were quantified by a solid phase radio-immunoassay (Charrière et al, 1988). Sera were diluted 1:50,000. Results were expressed as percentage of binding of total radioactivity (B/T %).

Statistical analysis: Values of weight and hindpaw volume were analysed for significance by Anova test. Clinical and radiological scales, and antibody response were analysed using the non-parametric Kruskall-Wallis and Mann-Whitney's U tests. The incidence of arthritis was analysed by chi-square test. The p significance level was 0.05.

RESULTS

The data obtained on day 32 are set out in table I.

1. Incidence of polyarthritis (systemic disease): Only 2/12 rats developed a polyarthritis in the control group (A) and 3/12 in IL-1 batch (C). This difference was not significant. In contrast, the incidence of the disease was significantly higher in MDP group (B) (11/12) as compared to the two other groups (p<0.001, chi square test).

2. Systemic disease: arthritic index - volume and X-ray scores of the left hindpaw: Only arthritic animals were taken into account to evaluate the severity of arthritis, i.e. 2, 11 and 3 rats in groups A, B and C respectively. The mean body weight decreased to a lesser extent in arthritic rats of the control group than in the others. Left hindpaw volume and arthritic index were not significantly different in arthritic animals of IL-1 group compared with those of control group. Diseased rats of the MDP group seemed to have a more intense polyarthritis though the differences were not significant except at the end of the study. On day 32, the radiological scores of the left hindpaw were also more severe, albeit not significantly, in arthritic rats of MDP group compared with those of IL-1 and control groups.

3. Time-course of the injected hindpaw lesions: All the rats were studied. The clinical score and the volume of the right injected hindpaw were significantly higher in group MDP than in the two other batches with an attenuation of these differences between day 7 and day 14. HrIL-1β had no pro-inflammatory action on the injected paw. The values of IL-1 group were even lower than those of the control group. The clinical score (mean ± S.E.M.) was significantly lower in IL-1 group compared to the control group either on day 15 (1.4 ± 0.9 and 2.3 ± 0.8, respectively) or on day 18 (1.8 ± 0.8 and 2.6 ± 0.7, respectively).

Group	Injected hindpaw		Noninjected paws (arthritic rats only)				Humoral response
	Volume (ml)	Clinical score (0-4)	Arthritic index (0-12)	Left hindpaw volume (ml)	X-ray scores (0-6) joint lesions	periost. reaction	B/T (%)
Control	2.87±0.43	2.3±0.6	1.5±0.7	1.85±0.07	0±0	0±0	35.5±10.2
MDP	3.60±0.55 (p<0.0003)	3.1±0.5 (p=0.002)	4.3±1.9 (p=0.04)	2.94±0.70 (p=0.05)	2.3±1.6 (NS)	1.8±1.3 (NS)	23.2±12.7 (p=0.02)
IL-1	2.75±0.48 (NS)	2.0±0.8 (NS)	2.3±1.2 (NS)	2.20±0.30 (NS)	1.3±0.6 (NS)	1.0±0 (NS)	10.1±8.9 (p<0.0001)

Table I. Clinical, radiological, and immunological data obtained on day 32 in MDP batch (hnCII + MDP) and IL-1 batch (hnCII + hrIL1ß) compared to control batch (hnCII). Results are expressed as mean ± SEM. Values of p≤0.05 were considered as significant (NS: non significant).

4. Humoral response to CII: The immune response to CII was surprisingly reduced (p=0.0001, Kruskall-Wallis test) in the IL-1 group compared with the two other batches (n=12 in each group). Antibody levels were also lower in the MDP group than in the control group (p=0.02). No correlation was found between the CII antibody level and the clinical or radiological parameters on day 32.

DISCUSSION

Since many adjuvant peptidoglycans act, at least partially, via the production of IL-1 (Vacheron et al, 1983), we hypothesized that MDP may have adjuvant properties in CIA through a local release of IL-1 by macrophages at the site of administration of the sensitizing emulsion. In our study, however, local administration of hrIL-1β simultaneously with collagen antigen did not worsen the disease. HrIL-1β had even an obvious attenuating action on humoral response to CII. This phenomenon was also noted, albeit less markedly, from day 14, on clinical parameters of the injected hindpaw.

These results might be explained by an increase of the clearance of the antigen. In fact, after the injection of the emulsion in the right hindpaw, the setting of specific immunitary response to hnCII needs a certain delay. IL-1 is chemotactic for leukocytes (Pettipher et al, 1986). When injected with the collagen emulsion, the cytokine may give an infiltration of leukocytes which might clear the antigen (hnCII) more rapidly (Jacobs et al, 1988) and, hence, decrease the specific antibody response to hnCII. Staruch and Wood (1983) demonstrated that IL-1 enhances in vivo secondary antibody responses in mice when it was given intraperitoneally 2 hours or more after the priming dose of antigen (bovine serum albumin). If IL-1 was injected at the same time as the antigen, they found a weak adjuvant effect while we had a decrease of type II collagen antibody in our experiment. This might be due to the different site of IL-1 injection.

Other pharmacological agents had been administered into the same site as the collagen antigen (Bober et al, 1985). Concanavalin A, pokeweed mitogen, tilorone, and even the phlogistic carrageenan might decrease the incidence of CIA probably through an effect on the immune system. It is noteworthy that these effects depended on the site of administration (i.e. local with the collagen emulsion or distant) and on the time at which the drugs were injected relative to the collagen injection.

In our experiment, the administration of IL-1 produced a favourable effect on the injected hindpaw (significant from day 15 to 18) and a decrease of CII antibody titer while it had no effect neither on the incidence nor on the severity of the systemic disease. The number of arthritic rats was however too small in IL-1 and control groups to conclude formally. An initial decrease of the amount of hnCII might explained the reduction of soft tissue inflammation of the right hindpaw and the diminution of the humoral response. The absence of correlation between anticollagen antibody production and clinical features (incidence and severity) reinforces the hypothesis of a multifactorial mechanism of the CII arthritogenicity. On the other hand, MDP greatly increased the incidence of the experimental arthritis. Clinical and radiological findings seemed also to be more severe than in the two others groups. This pejorative influence of MDP was not associated with an increase of humoral response to CII.

Finally, hrIL-1β (0.2 μg) did not exert adjuvant properties in CIA when injected simultaneously with hnCII. IL-1 might increase the collagen clearance which resulted in a decrease in humoral response and less severe clinical lesions of the injected hindpaw.

REFERENCES

Bober,L.A., Tivey,L.C., DaFonseca,M., Smith,S.R. and Watnick,A.S. (1985). Inhibition of collagen II arthritis by simultaneous administration of concanavalin A and other substances with antigen emulsion *Immunopharmacology* **9**, 97-107.

Charriere,G., Hartmann,D.J., Vignon,E., Ronzière,M.C., Herbage,D. and Ville,G. (1988). Antibodies to type I, II, IX and XI collagen in the serum of patients with rheumatic diseases. *Arthritis Rheum.* **31**, 325-332.

Fener,P., Bannwarth,B., Gillet,P., Netter,P., Regent,D., Pourel,J. and Gaucher,A. (1990). Influence of sulfasalazine on established collagen arthritis in rats. *Clin. Exp. Rheum.* **8**, 167-170.

Gillet,P., Bannwarth,B., Charrière,G., Leroux,P., Fener,P., Netter,P., Hartmann,D.J., Péré,P. and Gaucher,A. (1989). Studies on type II collagen induced arthritis in rats: an experimental model of peripheral and axial ossifying enthesopathy. *J. Rheumatol.* **16**, 721-728.

Jacobs,C., Young,D., Tyler,S., Callis,G., Gillis,S., Conlon,P.J. (1988). In vivo treatment with IL-1 reduces the severity and duration of antigen-induced arthritis in rats. *J. Immunol.* **141**, 2967-2974.

Koga,T., Sakamoto,S., Onoue,K., Kotani,S., Sumiyoshi,A. (1980). Efficient induction of collagen arthritis by the use of a synthetic muramyl dipeptide. *Arthritis Rheum.* **23**, 993-997.

Pettipher,E.R., Higgs,G.A. and Henderson,B. (1986). Interleukin 1 induces leukocyte infiltration and cartilage proteoglycan degradation in the synovial joint. *Proc. Natl. Acad. Sci. USA* **83**, 8749-8753.

Staruch,M.J. and Wood,D.D. (1983). The adjuvanticity of interleukin 1 in vivo. *J. Immunol.* **130**, 2191-2194.

Vacheron,F., Guenounou,M. and Neuciel,C. (1983). Induction of interleukin-1 secretion by adjuvant active peptidoglycans. *Infect. Immun.* **42**, 1049-1054.

AAS 32
Drugs in Inflammation

INFLUENCE OF AZELASTINE ON IL-1β GENERATION IN VITRO AND IL-1β-INDUCED EFFECT IN VIVO

U. Werner, J. Schmidt and I. Szelenyi

Department of Pharmacology, ASTA Pharma AG, Weismüllerstraße 45, D-6000 Frankfurt/Main, FRG

SUMMARY

The effects of the novel antiasthmatic/antiallergic compound azelastine on IL-1β were investigated in vitro and in vivo. In leukocytes both, intra- and extracellular IL-1 generation stimulated by LPS was inhibited dose dependently. In contrast azelastine did not prevent IL-1β-induced immigration of PMNs into the mouse ear. These findings suggest that azelastine is not an IL-1 antagonist but inhibits IL-1 synthesis and/or release in leukocytes.

INTRODUCTION

Interleukin 1 (IL-1), which is produced by monocytes/macrophages and by several other cell types has been demonstrated to mediate a variety of biological activities thought to be important in immunoregulation and immunopathology (Dinarello 1984). A wide variety of biological properties including fever production, T-cell activation and involvement in onset and development of inflammatory and immune reactions is attributed to IL-1. Since the late phase reaction of the asthmatic response is characterized by airway inflammation the therapeutic properties of antiasthmatic drugs should also include anti-inflammatory potentials. The novel long-acting antiasthmatic/antiallergic drug azelastine (4-(p-chlorobenzyl)-2(hexahydro-

1-methyl-1H-azepin-4-yl)-1-(2H)-phthalazinone hydrochloride) has been shown to have suppressive effects on the formation and action of various inflammatory mediators like histamine (Chand et al. 1985), leukotrienes (Achterrath-Tuckermann et al. 1988) and oxygen-derived radicals(Schmidt et al. 1990a).

In the present study we have examined the effect of azelastine on IL-1β generation in vitro and on IL-1ß action in a mouse-inflammation model.

MATERIALS AND METHODS

In vitro studies: Human blood was obtained from adult healthy volunteers by venepuncture using EDTA-vacutainer tubes (Sarstedt, FRG). After dextran (T 500, Pharmacia LKB, Sweden) sedimentation the resulting cells were washed twice in phosphate buffered saline (PBS) and resuspended to 4 x 10^6 cells/ml RPMI-medium (Boehringer Mannheim, FRG). Cell suspensions (0.1 ml) were transferred in a tissue culter plate.

azelastine was dissolved as a stock solution in pyrogen-free aqua bidestillata and subsequent dilutions were made in RPMI. Before adding lipopolysaccharides (LPS, from Escherichia coli, Sigma, FRG) in a final concentration of 100 ng/ml leukocytes were incubated with prewarmed drug solutions for 30 minutes.

After further 14 hours incubation at 37°C IL-1β content in the supernatant and in the cell lysate respectively was determined by ELISA (Quantikine™, R&D Systems, USA).

In vivo studies: Male NMRI mice (Savo, FRG) weighing 20-25g were injected subcutaneously with 150 U human recombinant IL-1β (Boehringer Mannheim, FRG) diluted in 20 μl phosphate-buffered saline (PBS) into the left ear. Control mice received the same volume of PBS. Mice were sacrificed 24 hours after IL-1 injection and both ears were removed and weighened (Maloff et al. 1989).

MPO is a marker enzyme for PMNs. The influx of PMNs into the inflamed tissue was estimated spectrometrically by determination of myeloperoxidase (MPO) activity according to Bradley et al. (1982). Ears were homogenized in a 50 mM potassium phosphate buffer, pH 6.0, containing 0.5% hexadecyltrimethylammonium bromide (Sigma, FRG), sonicated for 10 sec, freeze-thawed 3 times to release the contents of the primary granules of the PMNs and sonicated again. The suspensions were centrifuged at 16,000 x g for 30 min and the supernatants assayed. 100 μl of the material to be measured was mixed with 1.4 ml phosphate buffer containing 0.334 mg/ml o-dianisidine dihydrochloride (Sigma, FRG) and 0.0005% hydrogen peroxide. The changes of absorbance was measured at 450 nm and the equivalent amounts of MPO per mg mouse ear were determined. The contralateral ear, not injected with IL-1β, was taken for control.

RESULTS

Influence of azelastine on IL-1β generation: As shown in Fig. 1 human leukocytes stimulated overnight with LPS produce a large amount of IL-1β, which is partly secreted into the supernatant. Controls without LPS-stimulation exhibit only very low IL-1β levels, indicating that the leukocyte cultures are not contaminated by endotoxin during cultivation procedure. In presence of 1, 5, and 10 μM azelastine the amount of extracellular secreted IL-1β (3, 8, and 36% inhibition) as well as the intracellular IL-1β (2, 17, and 40% inhibition) is dose dependently decreased (Fig. 1). There was no crossreactivity by azelastine with the IL-1β ELISA (data not shown).

Influence of azelastine on IL-1β-induced tissue PMN immigration: Azelastine was not able to inhibit IL-1-induced PMN influx into the mouse ear. After oral treatment with 20 mg/kg azelastine 2 hours prior to the IL-1β injection there was a significant increase in MPO activity from 665 ± 150 to 1984 ± 169 nU/mg ear (+198%) in the inflamed ears compared to the control ears. Without azelastine MPO activity in the untraeted ear was 463 ± 117 nU/mg tissue. Injection of 150 U IL-1β resulted in 1592 ± 303 nU MPO/mg ear. This was an increase of 244% over the control ears. Pretreatment with 20 mg/kg p.o. 24 hours before followed by 2 mg/kg azelastine p.o. 2 hours prior to IL-1 injection resulted in a significant increase from 573 ± 124 to 1628 ± 407 nU/mg (+184%) in left to right ear. Compared to 201% increase (509 ± 19 to 1531 ± 273 nU MPO/mg tissue) in the vehicle-treated control group there was also no inhibition of IL-1 induced PMN immigration into the inflammation area (Fig. 2).

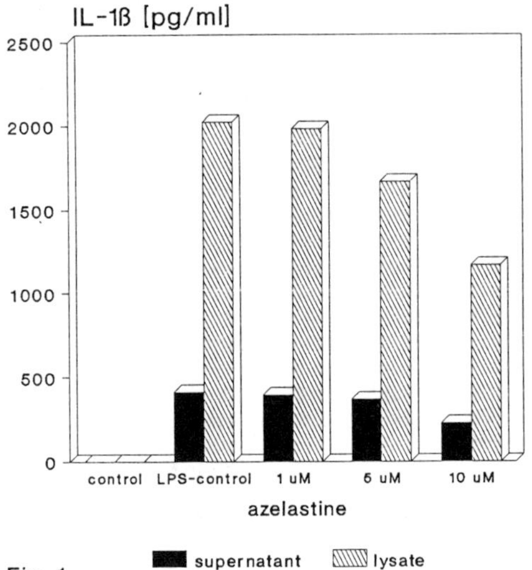

Fig. 1

LPS-induced IL-1β stimulation in human leukocytes, incubation: 14h with 100 ng/ml LPS

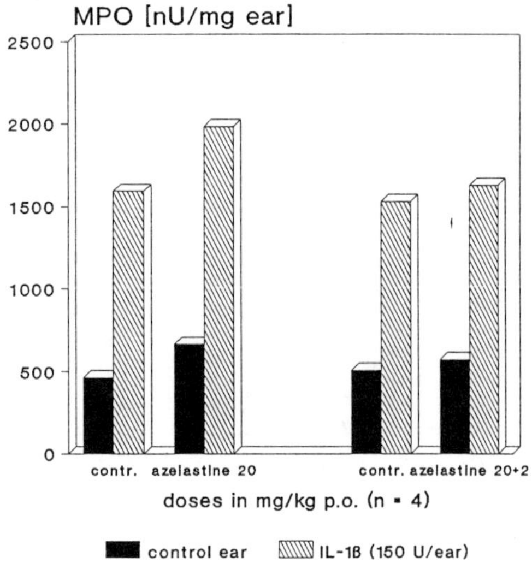

Fig. 2

Male NMRI mice(20-25 g),IL-1β injected s.c. 24h before determination of MPO, azelastine was administered resp. 2h and 24 plus 2h prior to IL-1

DISCUSSION

The present data demonstrate that azelastine decreases the LPS induced IL-1ß generation in human leukocytes. This effect may be related to the suggested interaction of azelastine with protein kinase C (Schmidt et al. 1990b), since Taniguchi et al. (1989) have shown that signal transduction pathway of LPS-induced IL-1β generation in human monocytes involves protein kinase C. Another mode of action of azelastine in this model may be based on its antileukotriene activity (Achterrath-Tuckermann et al. 1988), since formation of leukotrienes also appears to provide a positive signal for cytokine synthesis.

Local injection of IL-1 into tissues results in rapid recruitment of leukocytes from the blood compartment. IL-1 itself is not directly chemotactic, but elicits leukocyte extravasation indirectly by changing the adhesive properties of endothelial cells and inducing production of chemotactic cytokines. Azelastine failed to inhibit IL-1β induced granulocyte accumulation in the mouse ear as shown for dexamethasone (Maloff et al. 1989).

Because IL-1 stimulates expression of genes and/or receptors for other cytokines (IL-2 through IL-9, TNF), reduction of IL-1 synthesis may contribute to antiinflammatory and antiallergic effects in the lung. We conclude that azelastine is not a IL-1 antagonist, but inhibits IL-1 synthesis and/or release. This may be important for the beneficial role of azelastine in asthma therapy.

REFERENCES

Achterrath-Tuckermann, U.; T. Simmet, W. Luck, I. Szelenyi and B. A. Peskar, Inhibition of cysteinyl-leukotriene production by azelastine and its biological significance. Agents and Actions 24, 217-223 (1988)

Bradley, P.P.; D.A. Priebat, R.D. Christensen and G. Rothstein, Measurement of cutaneous inflammation: Estimation of neutrophil content with an enzyme marker. J. Invest. Dermatol. 78, 206-209 (1982)

Chand, N.; J. Pillar, W. Diamantis and R. D. Sofia, Inhibition of IgE-mediated allegic histamine release from rat peritoneal mast cells by azelastine and selected antiallergic drugs. Agents and Actions 16, 318-322 (1985)

Dinarello, C. A., Interleukin-1. Rev. Infect. Dis. 6, 51-95 (1984)

Maloff, B.L.; J.E. Shaw and T.M. Di Meo, IL-1 dependent model of inflammation mediated by neutrophils. J. Pharmacol. Meth. 22, 133-140 (1989)

Schmidt, J. and I. Szelenyi, Inhibition of guinea-pig alveolar macrophage superoxide anion generation by azelastine. Br. J. Pharmacol. 99 (Suppl.), 188P (1990a)

Schmidt, J.; B. Kaufmann, R. Lindstaedt and I. Szelenyi, Inhibition of chemiluminescence in granulocytes and alveolar macrophages by azelastine. Agents and Actions (1990b) in press)

Taniguchi, H.; T. Sakano, T. Hamasaki, H. Kashiwa and K. Ueda, Effect of protein kinase C inhibitor (H-7) and calmodulin antagonist (W-7) on pertussis toxin-induced IL-1 production by human adherent monocytes. Comparison with lipopolysaccharide as stimulator of IL-1 production. Immunology 67, 210-215 (1989)

SUBJECT INDEX